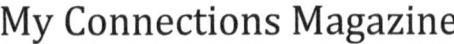 

Table of Contents:

**On the cover**: Connections Magazine Summer 2014

**Inside:** Societal trends are trends that relate to the social and cultural values and practices within a society.

**Feature story**: Who is your friend?

Page 15

Amazing Place must visit

Page 91

-Contents-

1-Fashion Body Talk Communication

My fashion statement connections:

Page 1-9

2-Health and Fitness

My diet connections:

Page 9-14

3-Social change and personal behaviors

My social connections

Page 21-25

4-Travel and Life Style

My favorite hang outs and travel places

Page 28-37

**HOW TO USE A SAUNA AND STEAM ROOM PROPERLY**

Page 92-95

<<<<<<<<<<<>>>>>>>>>>>
Food: L.A Times Jonathan Gold's choices for 14 of the most essential places to try.

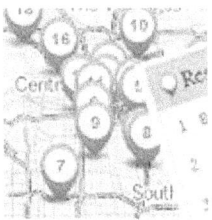

Gold's best Mexican restaurants My Connections:

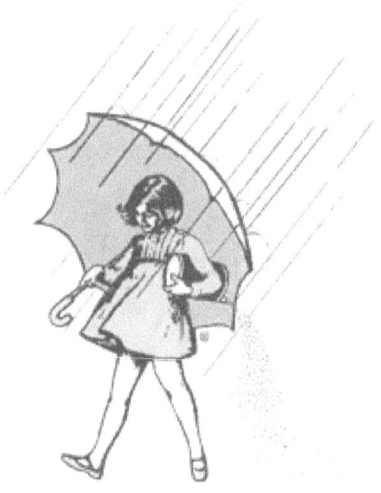

Facts are we are what we wear. Look Cowboy.

Every girl is looking for a well dressed man.

Make a statement again, this time is about:

You are trying to get our attention to support you

to help free American jailed journalist Austin Tice in Syria. For details information go to rsf.org (http://en.rsf.org/) for reporters without borders web and look up Austin Tice. In brief, on August 13, 2012, two days after his 31st birthday, Austin disappeared as he was preparing to travel from Daraya, near Damascus, Syria, to Beirut, Lebanon. He is

2

alive and he is not held by ISIS.

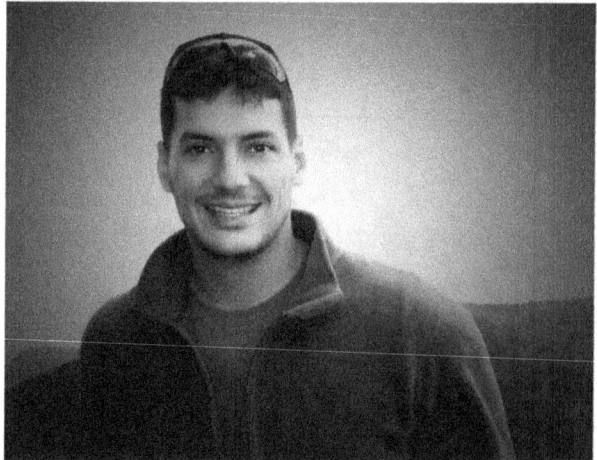

Syria is the world's most dangerous country for journalists since the start of the uprising in March 2011, with hundreds of journalists and citizen-journalists arrested, kidnapped or killed by the various parties involved in the conflict, as Reporters Without Borders reported constantly. The local journalists have especially paid a high price in their fight for freedom of information.,With everything relevant to the situation make a statement.

# REPORTERS WITHOUT BORDERS
## FOR FREEDOM OF INFORMATION

Source and Credit to Reporters Without borders. (rsf mean reporters without borders in French: reporters sans frontiers).
MCM Managing Editor EddieAdel.

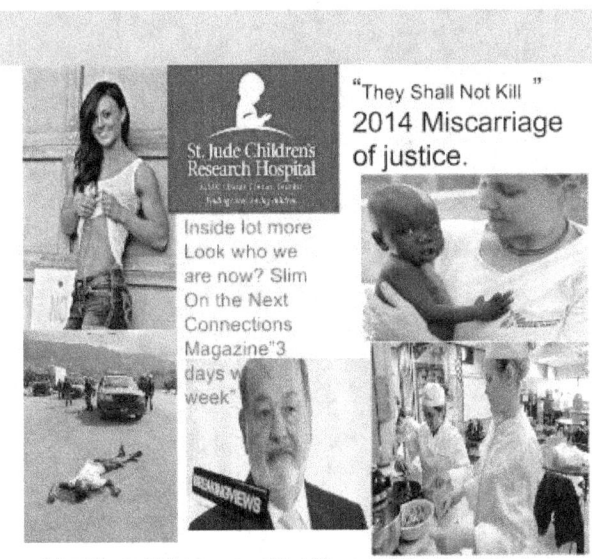

"They Shall Not Kill"
2014 Miscarriage of justice.

Inside lot more Look who we are now? Slim On the Next Connections Magazine"3 days w week"

Give the gift that save life. To serve and protect........

MCM last issue cover: Nov, Dec, Jan. 2014-2015

## THIS FASHION STATEMENT IS FOR YOU: YOU ARE WHAT YOU WEAR: FASHION, CLOTHING, AND COSTUME

– by Brittany Janiece Foster (B.F.A., '09)

The clothes we wear mean something to us as well as to the people who see us. Clothing changes the way we move and feel. How different do your feet feel when you wear high heels or tennis shoes? Flip flops or lace-up boots? How different do you feel in your favorite flannel pajama

pants and worn t-shirt rather than a tuxedo?

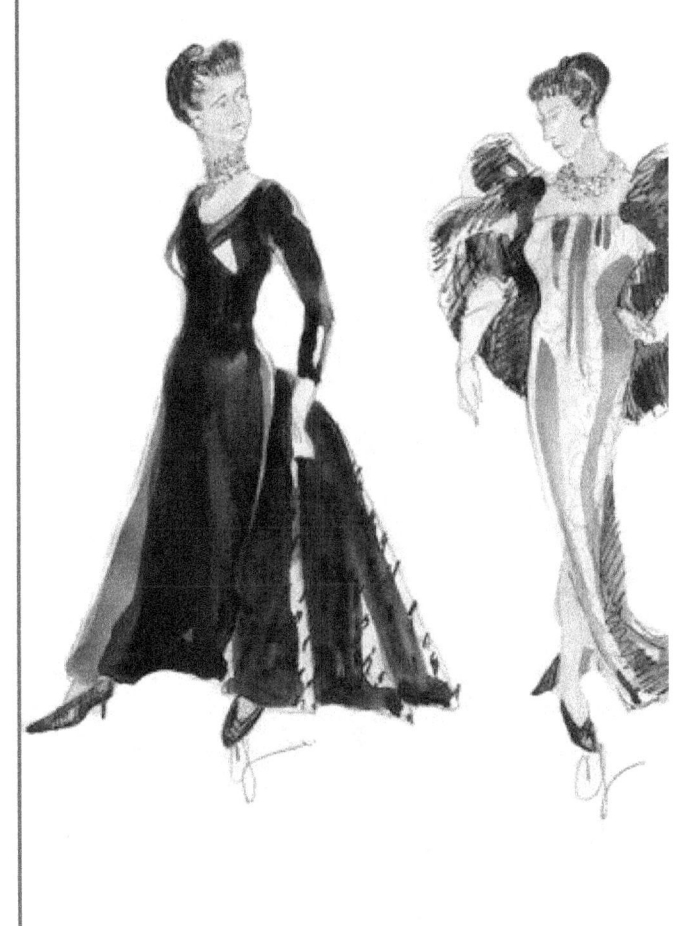

by Claudia J. Stevens for *La Discreta Enamorada* 2006

3

Fashion helps us to define our individual self. It also aids us in presenting a certain kind of persona to the outside world. The clothes we wear every day are different from haute couture fashion and from theatrical costumes. While high fashion and costumes help the wearer project a certain image, the reasons we choose any of the three are very specific. The clothes we wear every day must be practical: they cover our body for warmth, modesty, and purpose. Self-expression is a by-product, often welcome but not necessary. Models wear a particular designer's fashions to demonstrate his or her creative talent. They may wear a designer's less comfortable garment only long enough to walk down the runway and back or in a photography session, but students going to school or business people, teachers, or construction workers likely want to dress in clothes they can wear all day and multiple times that are suited to the tasks of their lives. These people will not want to worry, for example, about ultra-wrinkly fabrics creasing every time they take a step or sit down during the day. Fashions, especially in haute couture, must be bigger and brighter than life, because designers want to make an artistic or aesthetic statement. In the same way, every day clothes would not be appropriate for the fashion runway, because most of us wear jeans to school or suits to work, neither of which makes much of a bold aesthetic statement—but which are comfortable and useful and express our personalities.

Costumes on the stage bridge the gap between the fashions on the runway and everyday clothing. If everyday clothing reflects our self-expression, then costume design reflects the creative expression of the combination of the designer and the production. Actors, like models and unlike the rest of us, usually don't get to choose what they wear or have a say in the design, beyond expressing difficulties in movement, breathing, or fit. Costumes, like fashion, seek to make a statement; costumes express the production and the play, while fashion expresses the creativity of the individual designer.

On the stage, it is usually necessary that the costumes be interesting to look at; however, actors have different physical and aesthetic demands than fashion models. Models need to be able to walk up and down the catwalk for a minute or two and make the haute couture fashion displayed (and thus the designer) look good, actors may need to be onstage for up to two or three hours, speaking and moving the entire time. The actor must be able to breathe comfortably, so that he or she can project the dialogue. Actors must be able to walk around the space, or crawl, dance, do jumping jacks, fight with a sword, or any number of other physical activities, so costumes must not hinder an actor's movement.

The costume designer's role in designing the clothing for a play is different from that of a fashion designer. A fashion designer considers only his or her ideas or, if making a gown for a specific customer, what that patron wants. Generally, the designer's line will be reproduced by manufacturers using his or her original ideas. On the other hand, a costume designer will design each costume in a production as a one-time only outfit, worn by a specific character and tailored to a specific actor's body. The costume designer cannot simply put costumes on the stage because they are pretty or well-made or came from his or her ideas about clothes. The costume designer must analyze the playwright's script in order to know the characters.

Costumes serve several specific purposes in the theatre beyond allowing the audience to identify each individual actor-character onstage. Such factors as the character's gender, age, and social status (old queen versus pageboy, for example) play into the design. The designer must also take into account a character's personality: is he or she extroverted or introverted, honest or deceitful, intelligent or stupid, conformist or freethinking: a rock star versus a librarian. Characters' differences should manifest in what they wear onstage so that the audience can see the difference.

Compare two characters from La Discreta Enamorada. In the first scene Belisa, a middle-aged widow, is clad in a simple, modest black dress that covers her from neck to toe, while Gerarda, a high-class escort, wears a fine, black lace dress with a nude underlay that hugs her body only to the knee. What do their costumes say about these characters? Belisa is old-fashioned, conservative, or modest; further, she does not spend money on frivolities like fancy clothing. Gerarda is rich enough to purchase fancy dresses and is less concerned with being "proper": the silhouette and material of her dress are meant to attract the eye and to reveal her body's shape. How do costumes give an indication of age? The lines of the costumes might help indicate a character's age to the audience. Most of Belisa's clothing probably include floor-length skirts and thus restrict the actress's movement—suggesting middle-age—while the clothes of Fenisa, her daughter, will have skirts that come to mid-calf and move more freely, which will convey her youth and vivacity.

Costumes also give clues to the audience about time period in which the play's production takes place. For example: a character clothed in a doublet and hose is probably not found in a play set in 1956, just as a character in jeans and a leather jacket is probably not in a play about 1776: if these costumes did appear in these time periods, there would be a good explanation for them. The designer must be especially thoughtful while creating costumes for same-aged actors, because two actors who play a father and son can be the same age, especially in college productions.

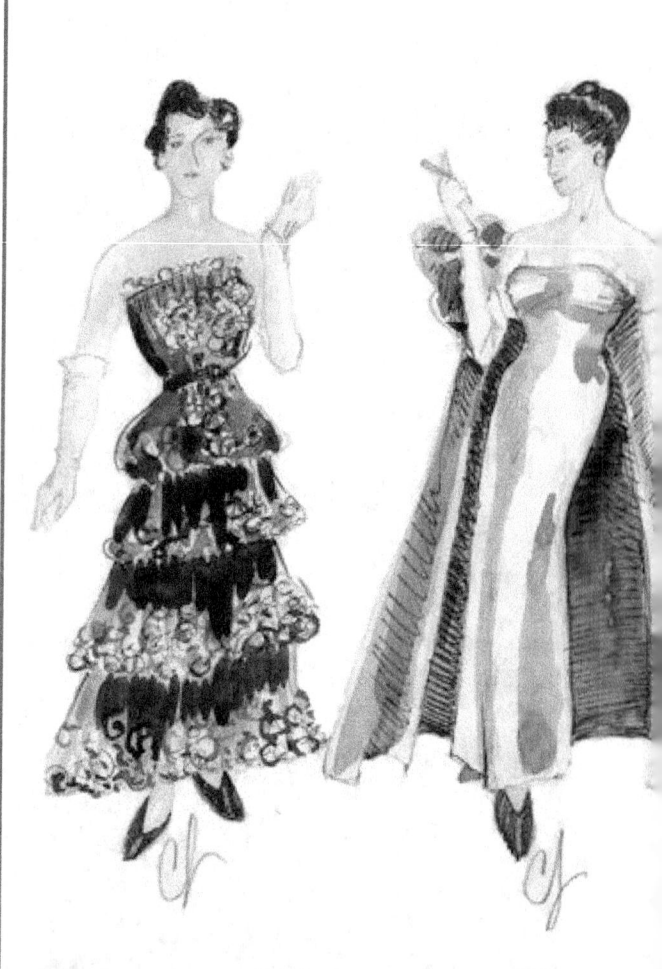

by Claudia J. Stevens for *La Discreta Enamorada* 2006

It is obvious that costumes are as important to the actors as they are to the audience. Just as our own clothes change us when we change roles in life, stage clothes can change a character.

Many times, actors will say that their character comes to life when they get into their costumes. It can make a huge different to an actress if she rehearses barefoot and then puts on stilettos, or in her own jeans and t-shirt but dons a corset for performances. Costumes are not just made up of clothes like shirts, pants, and dresses, but include shoes, hats, wigs, masks, makeup, and accessories such as glasses, jewelry, fans, handkerchiefs, handbags, pocket watches, and scarves. All these items are things an actor can use to help create the character and are usually selected for the actor by the costume designer. An actor might discover that when he puts on his character's glasses, the character tries to hide behind them or when he puts on a pair of boots, the character may use the loud sound they make to command attention.

The costume design must also collaborate with other creative artists of the production. The costume designer, the light designer, and the set designer must all meet with the director to interpret the play and to form one vision of their particular production of the play. The costume designs must fit in with the design of the rest of the show. Together, they must all create one coherent picture, based primarily on the playwright's text and the director's vision. It would be inappropriate to have all the characters wearing silk gowns in a play that takes place in a prison. If the designers never met to discuss the overall design, the production would be a disaster because all the components must work together and contribute to the whole. For example, costumers and lighting designers must work together because when different colors of light hit certain colors of fabric, the lights can change the color of the fabric; the lighting can change the reflective quality or wash out a color. If a costume designer creates a lovely green gown, a lighting designer could not put a red light on it or it would look a muddy brownish color, and all the work the costumer carefully put into that dress would be wasted. The same is true if there are several characters onstage wearing several different bright colors. The costumer and lighting designer must ensure that all the colors can work together to create a coherent picture onstage.

Claudia Stephens is the costume designer for La Discreta Enamorada and an associate professor in the Division of Theatre at SMU. For this production of Lope de Vega's play, she has based her designs on those of the 20th-century Spanish fashion designer, Cristobal Balenciaga: this is because the SMU production of this is because the SMU production of La Discreta Enamorada is set in Spain during the 1950s, but in the late 16th-century when de Vega wrote it. Balenciaga designed many gowns with interesting shapes, like layers of puffy balloon skirts and voluminous sleeves shaped like Chinese lanterns, made of expensive fabrics like black silks. How does Stephens use Balenciaga's designs to create costumes for the show? She kept the architectural shapes used by the designer as the foundation for her costumes. The costumes in this production will still have the visually stimulating silhouettes but will be modified so that the actors can still dance and move freely about the stage without bulky sleeves or skirts getting in their way. Additionally, the costumes must be constructed with a budget in mind; a college production will not support using the same expensive materials Balenciaga used.

Fashion, everyday clothing, and costume each demonstrate creative expression. Without them, life would be bland. The next time you are watching a play or a movie, think about how the costumes you see inform you about the characters. The next time you see a photograph of a model in haute couture fashion, think about what that designer is telling us about her or his artistic vision. The next time you choose clothing for school or work, consider the messages you are sending by the silhouette, fabric, fit, and color of your clothing: it does a lot more than just keep you warm.

Let your body talk, yes body language is very important and is slightly different than "fashion statement'.

How is body language different from fashion statement?

From facial expressions to adjusting posture or postures movement overall the impression is obvious to send first, second, third, and unlimited perceptions.

We got too far but not too far too get confused. We are about fashion statement, trying to cover body language, and the combination to include impressions and perceptions.

Fashion statement 2015 is cold hot warm and yes windy too.

Change in climate is making huge difference all over the world in how we continue to live and act every day. Cold winter made almost everyone to double up on clothing to stay warm.

To step by step cover the advance subjects of body language, impressions, and perceptions:

Smile and you show happy face accepting what is offered from everything around you. Happiness is a body language sing of accepting, agree to what is going on, relax and want more. Eye contact is another sign of body language and it can be a sign of happiness or sadness. How about the most international sign of body language, not the middle finger sign?

But nodding your head down for yes, or it is ok, accepting sign, and nodding the head up is a sign of no, negative, and disagree too.

Posture is often use by professionals to show energy is up by standing vertical as possible which mean healthy look as a positive sign to accept or move forward with whatever subject in progress to deal with, and it can make or break the camel back too.

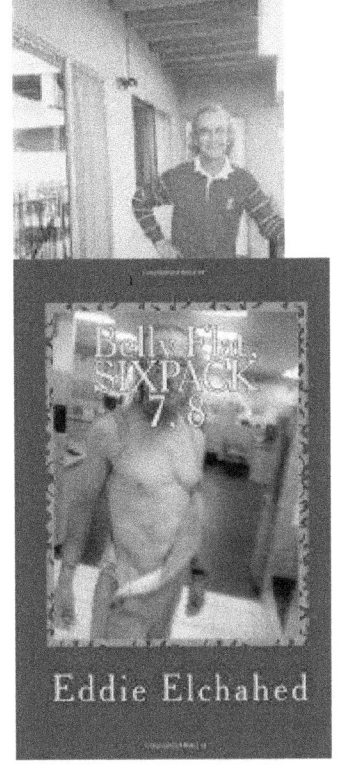

Eddie Elchahed

Perception and first impression are crucial to open up any door sort of speak. Perception at first look can last forever if either positive or negative. It is very important to be perceived as set to be or otherwise to change that perception could be impossible. Perception, perception , and perception is worth lot more than: Location , location, and as they make it look in real estate location.

There are three components to perception according to a Wikipedia scholar:

1. The Perceiver, the person who becomes aware about something and comes to a final understanding. There

9

are 3 factors that can influence his or her perceptions: experience, motivational state and finally emotional state. In different motivational or emotional states, the perceiver will react to or perceive something in different ways. Also in different situations he or she might employ a "perceptual defence" where they tend to "see what they want to see".

2. The Target. This is the person who is being perceived or judged. "Ambiguity or lack of information about a target leads to a greater need for interpretation and addition."

3. The Situation also greatly influences perceptions because different situations may call for additional information about the target.

Weconnect2.com publishing and digital network home to Law Enforcement Community Interface. Ask a cop: Police Without Borders on the world wide web.
policewithoutborders.com

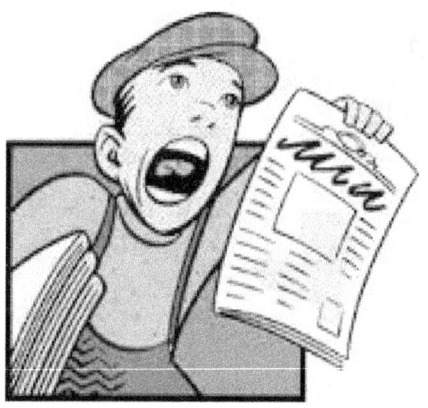

Perception is everything from your fashion statement , body language, impression, and timing. Let timing be our topic in the next issue.

What is first impression? It is different than perception by making an impression is moving forward to apply oneself in a specific matter adjusted to the situation. Good or bad impression can last a short time in comparison to perception. We are often perceived by others, but we make impression to others.

What is most important of none verbal communication techniques?

We can argue forever with pros and cons and on both sides of the argument there are the benefits of one more than the other, but we must all come to the final motion to agree that fashion statement win for generally can be use by everyone.

Making a fashion statement it can be slightly clear than body language, and it is easily perceived fast and with high percentage close to target than other means of communications skills, and the overall impression can fade immediately to focus on the correct statement.

# Health and Fitness

My diet connections:

Diet tips. Food and liquid for diabetes.

Diabetes type 2.

Type 2 Diabetes: What Is It?

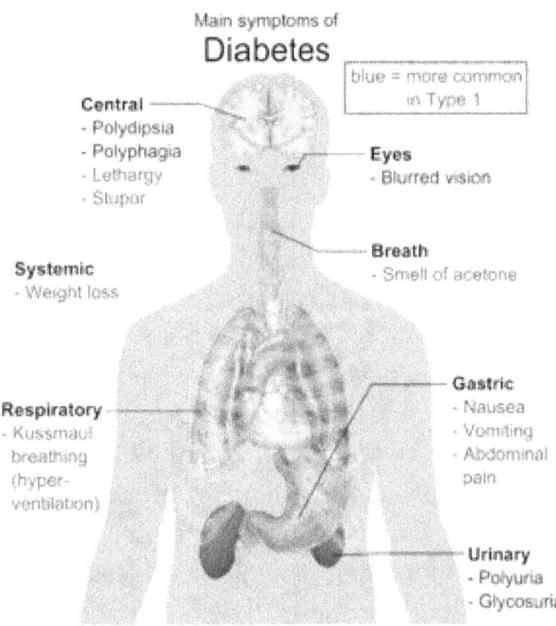

Main symptoms of
**Diabetes**

blue = more common in Type 1

**Central**
- Polydipsia
- Polyphagia
- Lethargy
- Stupor

**Eyes**
- Blurred vision

**Systemic**
- Weight loss

**Breath**
- Smell of acetone

**Respiratory**
- Kussmaul breathing (hyper-ventilation)

**Gastric**
- Nausea
- Vomiting
- Abdominal pain

**Urinary**
- Polyuria
- Glycosuria

Often ignored or treated with careless approach it become a much dangerous blood sugar disease than the normal insulin treated Type 1 diabetes.

Many diabetics with type 2 are not coached about their proper diet. Considering the more information available about diabetes type 1, most people ignore the details information about diabetes type 2.

Diet is the number one factor in both diabetes diseases type 1, and type 2. Food intake is very important to the blood stream including any liquid intake, proper rest as well, and taking medications as prescribed by physicians.

This issue we focus on processed food. Many don't know what is processed foods, how is it cooked, where is it cooked, and how to avoid eating processed food.

Why take any chance with it, processed food, let us consider all processed food is not healthy for any diabetes.

Funny it is never called processed food, and often glamorized with the taste, the price, and the value for so much on your dollar compare to other products. True many processed food is tasty and for the price it become lot more tasty than other food such as fresh meat, vegetables, and fruit.

This is my approach to the lack of knowledge about processed food for people with diabetes type 2. It is to make sure that we pass on the words to them by all means possible, keeping in mind that there are plenty of sources on the web to help them.

Here are Los Angles Times restaurant critic Jonathan Gold's choices for 14 of the most essential places to try.

Claudia Stephens is the costume designer for La Discreta Enamorada and an associate professor in the Division of Theatre at SMU. For this production of Lope de Vega's play, she has based her designs on those of the 20th-century Spanish fashion designer,

Cristobal Balenciaga: this is because the SMU production of **1. Babita:** One of the most serious Mexican restaurants on the Eastside, a casual corner joint whose service is burnished to a white-tablecloth sheen. Chef-owner Roberto Berrelleza is especially gifted at the cuisine of his hometown of Los Mochis on the Sinaloa coast. 1823 S. San Gabriel Blvd., San Gabriel, (626) 288-Claudia Stephens is the costume designer for La Discreta Enamorada and an associate professor in the Division of Theatre at SMU. For this production of Lope de Vega's play, she has based her designs on those of the 20th-century Spanish fashion designer, Cristobal Balenciaga: this is because the SMU production of ee-Press-Release.com/ -- Preventing weak abdominal tissues is first step to avoid a ""Hernia""…..I'am sure more than enough information available about the hernia. Specific details how to prevent a hernia are limited due to the complication in predicting when a muscle tissue become so weak to break or pup-up. It is almost like the muscle cramp.

Basically a weak tissue of a muscle, 75 % of hernia are in the abdominal wall, some in the groin area. more men than women have it. It is a displacement of an organ when spaces become too tight , sort of speak, the push come to shuv and where is weakness in the muscle tissuee(usualyin the lower Abs) a bulged pup-out.

Severe abdominal hernia can be extremely dangerous. Thus, it cut off the blood supply to the muscle eliminating the flow of oxygen. This type of hernia(severe abdominal hernia) normal in the lower abdomen need immediate surgery because of the extreme pain one can endure while the oxygen is not carried to the muscle through the blood supply.

Applying presure to the bulged spot(the hernia) as it occure will reduce tremendous amount of pain.

13

Many think it is over since 95% of the pain will vanish due to pup-back of the bulged hernia spot.

A severe hernia need an immediate emergency surgery procedure. The bulged area will return with the same extreme amount of pain without any prior signs and no specific time line.

If you had a (fixed) abdominal hernia, it is best to consult a physician before participating in any form of weight loss program, fitness routine, and any exercise regimen.

it is almost impossible to predict a weakness in the abdominal muscle tissues. Therefore, strengthening the abdominal muscles wall is one of the many forward steps in preventing any weak tissues.

Cardio exercise and weight loss food diet are definitely some of the best answers to maintaining intenstants

and organs from pushing through
anywhere in your body beside the
Abs tissues, weak or strong.

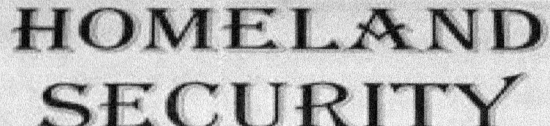

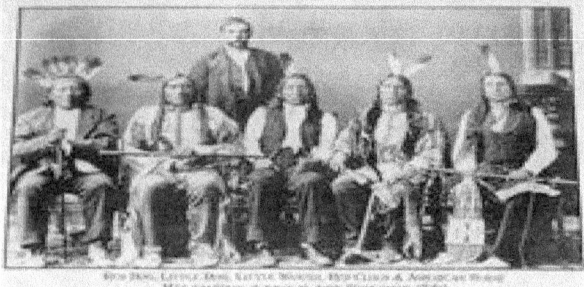

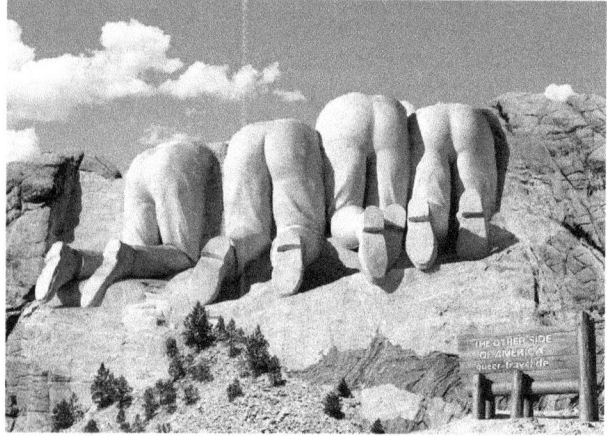

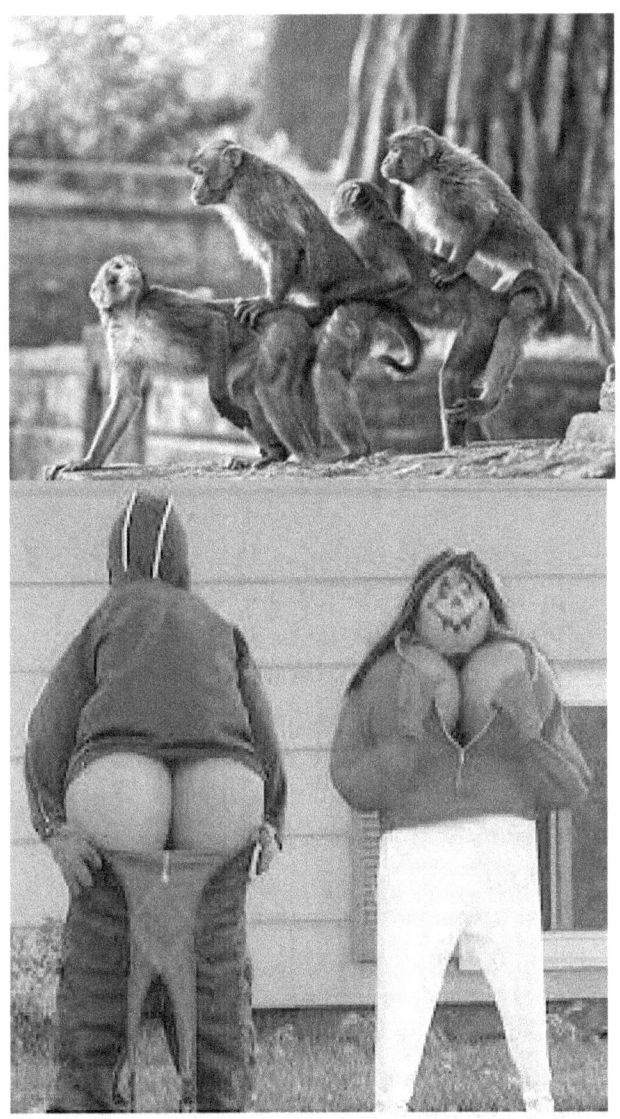

www.iLikeitFunny.com

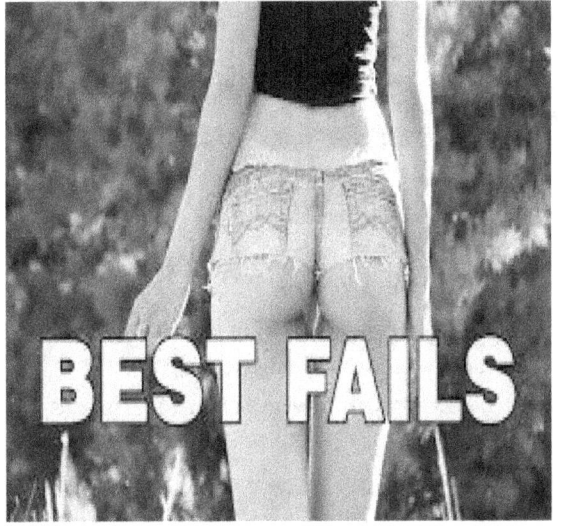

Funny
Photos

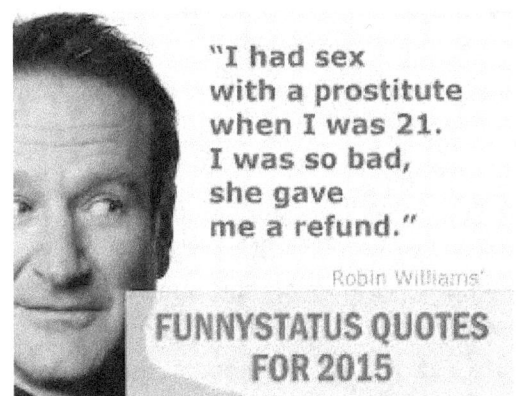

"I had sex
with a prostitute
when I was 21.
I was so bad,
she gave
me a refund."

Robin Williams'

FUNNYSTATUS QUOTES
FOR 2015

Feature Story

# Feature Story

### Who is your friend?

Once in a while we ought to veer from animated politico-cultural issues, so let us discuss the issue of friendship in this piece. Determining what characteristics a friend should possess is quite a daunting task, but learning from one another – via a compendium of both heartwarming and heartbreaking stories – can be helpful, even as we go about our daily lives. So, who or what is a friend? A friend could be many things: someone who sticks closer than a brother; someone who looks out for your wellbeing; someone who accepts your strengths and weaknesses unquestioningly; someone who rejoices with you when something good happens in your life, like a promotion at work or the birth of a child; someone who mourns with you when you experience tragedy, and so on.

Generally, however, you may only know a true friend when difficulties come your way: when you are sick and need someone to nurse you back to sound health, when you are out of work and need some money, when you have lost your home and need a place to rest your head temporarily, when you need a helping hand to deal with the avalanche of life's problems.

While a student at Accra Academy a little

over two decades ago, James lost his lover to his best friend, Peter, just because James did not own a video player and color television (great items to own at that time!) – and Peter did! Unknown to James at the time, Peter, who secretly coveted James' girlfriend, was able to lure the lady to his place to watch movies, and when the lady realized that James did not have the wherewithal to purchase such entertainment gadgets, she allowed Peter to seduce her. Some will be quick to blame the girl because, after all, she allowed herself to fall for Peter, but can we really justify Peter's behavior and blame it all on the girl? A friend just does not do what Peter did! After all, there were so many other single girls in Accra at the time, so why did Peter take his best friend's lover? A few years ago, while a student at the University of Ghana, Legon, a guy seduced his professed best friend's girlfriend, resulting in a prolonged affair – and the original boyfriend would not know for a very long time that he and his nefarious pal were both drinking from the same fountain of pleasure! Some may want to, once again, blame this particular girl entirely, but I believe that a greater portion of the blame should be placed squarely on the shoulders of the devious guy, for it is wrong to seek the lover of a bosom friend. In fact, the aforementioned imprudent behavior simply breaks the rules of conventionalism!

A friend is someone who wishes others

well, especially those closest to him or her. If you have a friend who shows little interest in your positive goals, just drop him or her. A friend is the husband who

............................................................

..

## Tex-Mex Chili

Hearty and spicy, this is a man's chili for sure. You can also simmer on the stove—the longer, the better! —Eric Hayes, Antioch, California

Read more: Claudia Stephens is the costume designer for La Discreta Enamorada and an associate professor in the Division of Theatre at SMU. For this production of Lope de Vega's play, she has based her designs on those of the 20th-century Spanish fashion designer, Cristobal Balenciaga: this is because the SMU production of

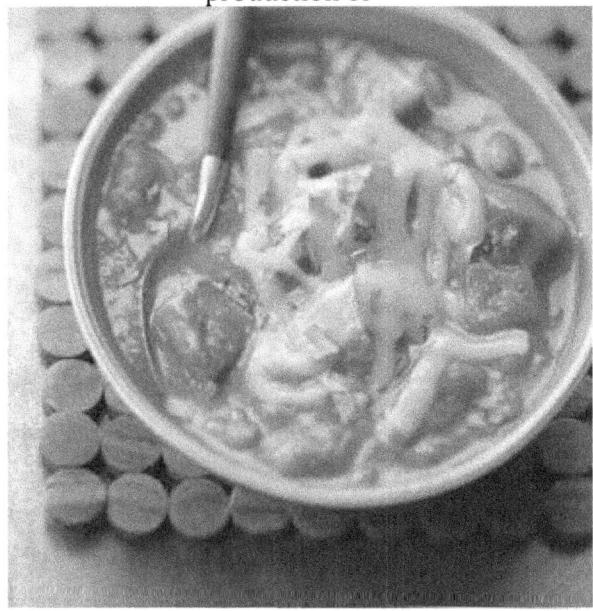

## Tex-Mex Chili

**Directions**

1. In a large skillet, brown beef in oil in batches. Add garlic; cook 1 minute longer. Transfer to a 6-qt. slow cooker.

STIR IN THE BEANS, TOMATO SAUCE, TOMATOES, WATER, TOMATO PASTE, SALSA VERDE AND SEASONINGS. COVER AND COOK ON LOW FOR 6-8 HOURS OR UNTIL MEAT IS TENDER. GARNISH EACH SERVING WITH CHEESE AND CILANTRO. YIELD: 12 SERVINGS (1-1/3 CUPS EACH).

ORIGINALLY PUBLISHED AS TEX-MEX CHILI IN TASTE OF HOME DECEMBER/JANUARY 2010, P26

READ MORE: CLAUDIA STEPHENS IS THE COSTUME DESIGNER FOR LA DISCRETA ENAMORADA AND AN ASSOCIATE PROFESSOR IN THE DIVISION OF THEATRE AT SMU. FOR THIS PRODUCTION OF LOPE DE VEGA'S PLAY, SHE HAS BASED HER DESIGNS ON THOSE OF THE 20TH-CENTURY SPANISH FASHION DESIGNER, CRISTOBAL BALENCIAGA: THIS

## IS BECAUSE THE SMU
## PRODUCTION OF INGREDIENTS

- 3 pounds beef stew meat

- 1 tablespoon canola oil

- 3 garlic cloves, minced

- 3 cans (16 ounces *each*) kidney beans, rinsed and drained

- 3 cans (15 ounces *each*) tomato sauce

- 1 can (14-1/2 ounces) diced tomatoes, undrained

- 1 cup water

- 1 can (6 ounces) tomato paste

- 3/4 cup salsa verde

- 1 envelope chili seasoning

- 2 teaspoons dried minced onion

- 1 teaspoon chili powder

- 1/2 teaspoon crushed red pepper flakes

- 1/2 teaspoon ground cumin

- 1/2 teaspoon cayenne pepper

- Shredded cheddar cheese and minced fresh cilantro

2.

**Read more**: Claudia Stephens is the costume designer for La Discreta Enamorada and an associate professor in the Division of Theatre at SMU. For this production of Lope de Vega's play, she has based her designs on those of the 20th-century Spanish fashion designer, Cristobal Balenciaga: this is because the SMU production of

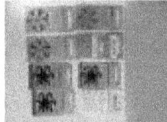

Claudia Stephens is the costume designer for La Discreta Enamorada and an associate professor in the Division of Theatre at SMU. For this production of Lope de Vega's play, she has based her designs on those of the 20th-century Spanish fashion designer, Cristobal Balenciaga: this is because the SMU production of

New list

Claudia Stephens is the costume designer for La Discreta Enamorada and an associate professor in the Division of Theatre at SMU. For this production of Lope de Vega's play, she has based her designs on those of the 20th-century Spanish fashion designer, Cristobal Balenciaga: this is because the SMU production of

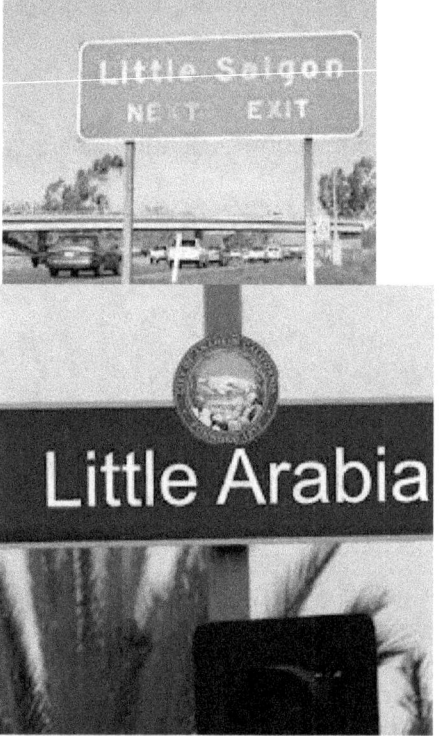
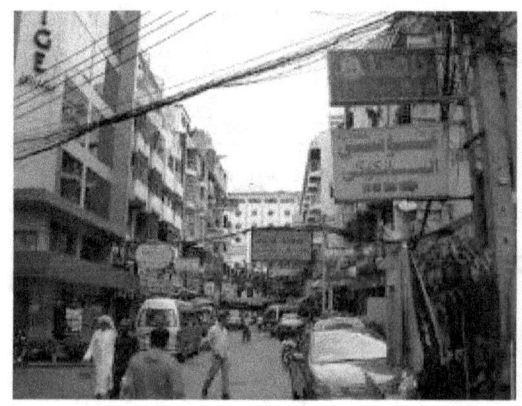
Claudia Stephens is the costume designer for La Discreta

Claudia Stephens is the costume designer

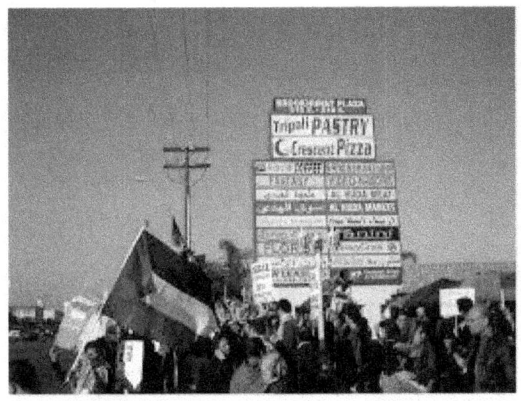

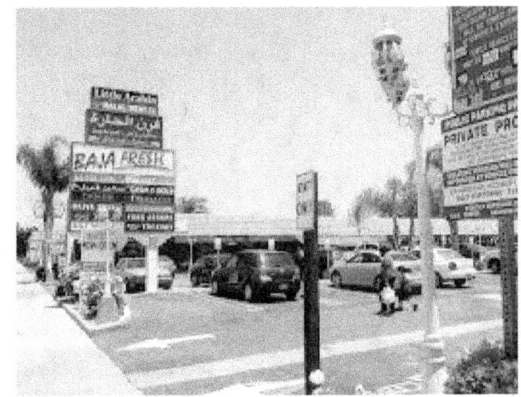

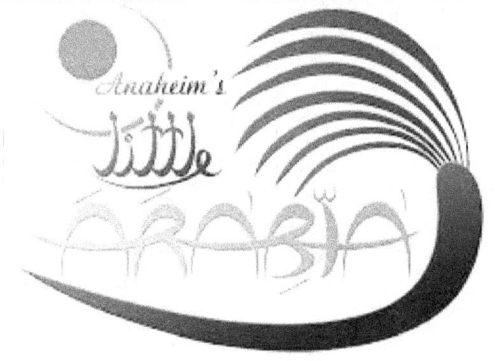

To order printed copy of My Connections Magazine: amazon.com search books MC Magazine or "CONNECTIONS MAGAZINE", FOR YOUR DIGITAL COPY GO TO IHUT the digital online store at nusjournal.com or newsusjournal.com.

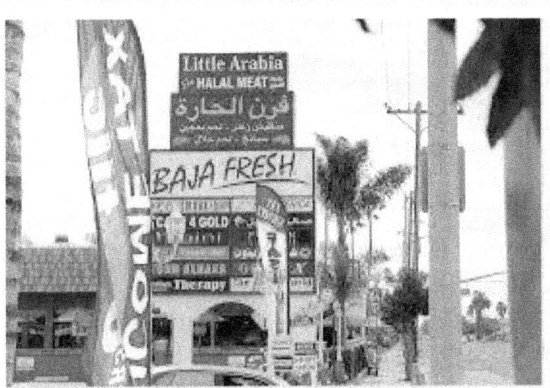

To order printed copy of My Connections Magazine: amazon.com search books MC Magazine or "CONNECTIONS MAGAZINE", FOR YOUR DIGITAL COPY GO TO IHUT the digital online store at nusjournal.com or newsusjournal.com.

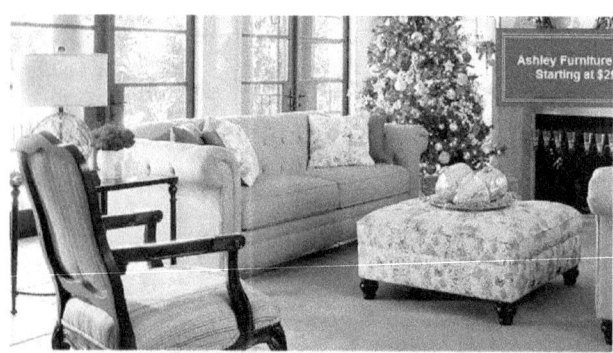
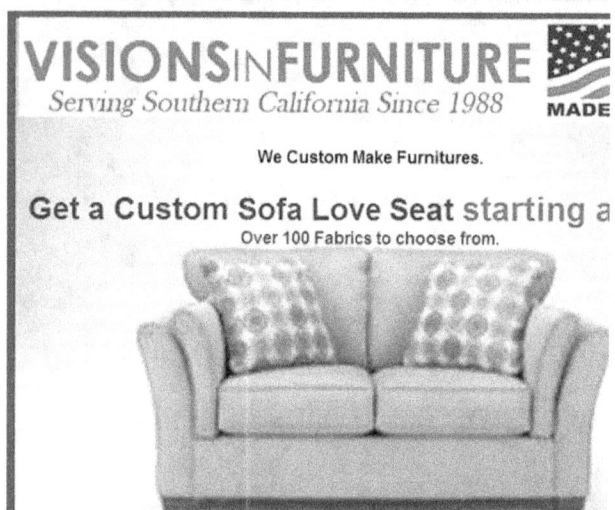
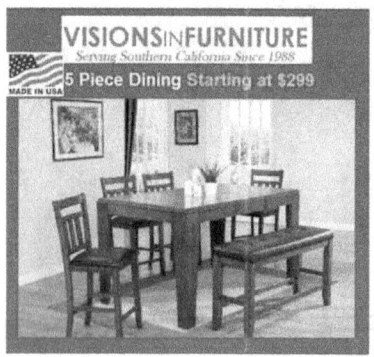
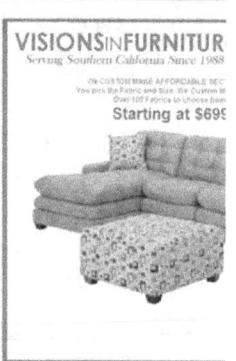
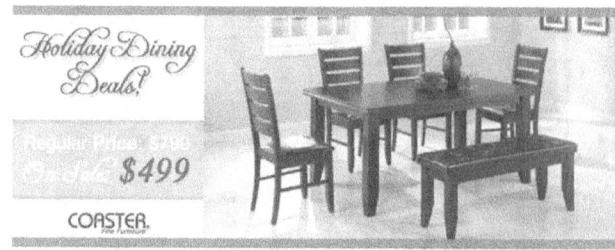
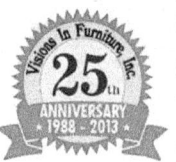
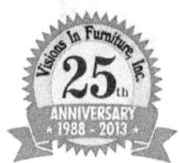
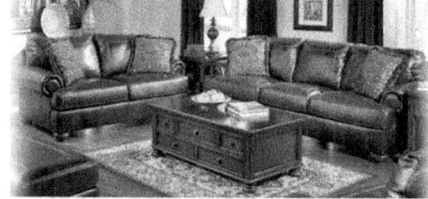
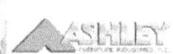
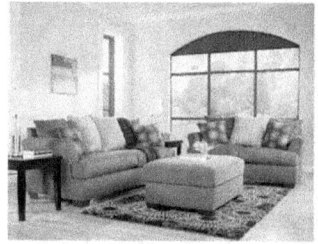
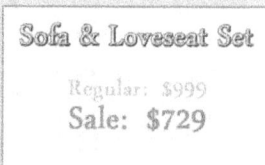
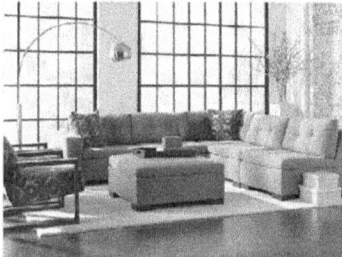

Visit on the web for more details and special offers.

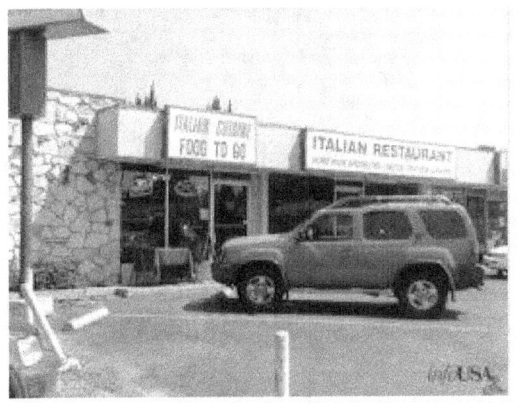

# Carolina:

Carolinaitalianrestaurant.com

For more information and details.

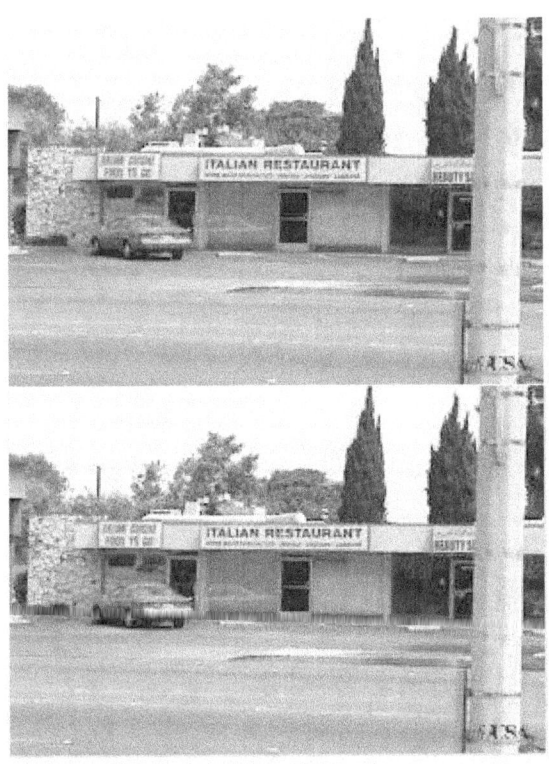

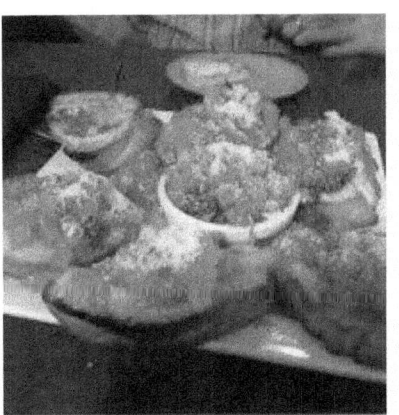

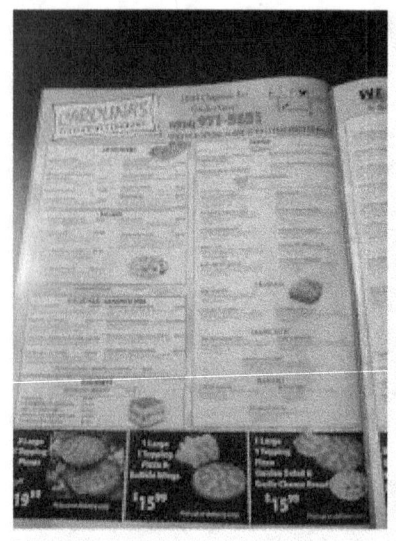

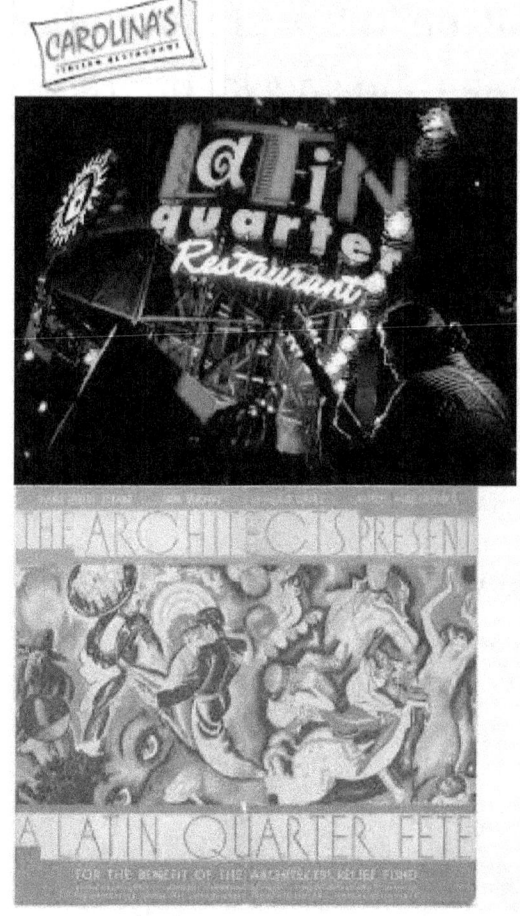

Little towns news provided on the world

wide web by News U.S. Journal. Tune in and browse at

## nusjournal.com

We are a blog of news articles, web contents, and most popular posts.

Also we are proud to be there for all the readers and audience for the past seven years at weconnect2.com publishing and digital network. We are here to stay. To provide the best

we can of related news articles to enhance our audience overall skills.

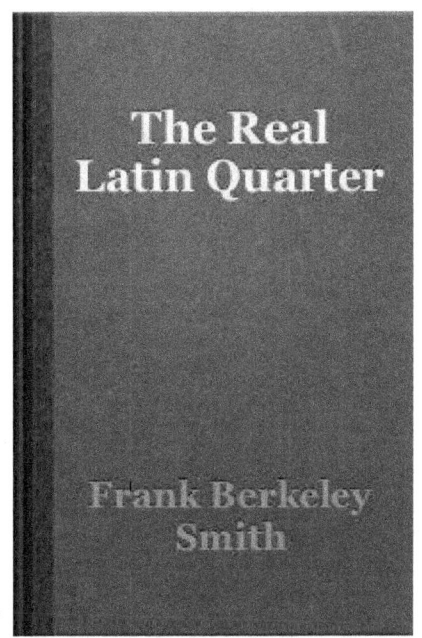

## SOCIETAL TRENDS

Societal trends are trends that relate to the social and cultural values and practices within a society. These are long term trends (at least two to five years) that explain why people behave the way they do. They are intergenerational. A few societal trends are only applicable to one specific group, but many of these effect society as a whole.

Some societal trends are caused by a single disruptive event (like 9/11), person (like Barack Obama) or technology (like the mobile phone). Other trends develop over the years – like a longing for 'real', as more and more aspects of life become fake or artificial. Most trends are interrelated and therefore overlap with others.

The TrendsActive societal trends are very practical and to-the-point and easy to incorporate into strategy, communication and product development.

## UNCERTAIN TIMES

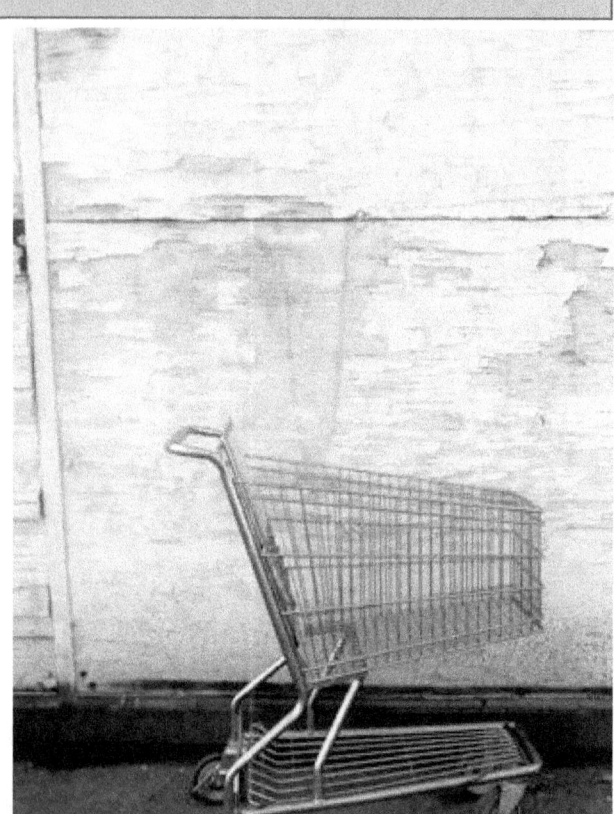

We live in uncertain times. Right now, we are suffering a recession. But in the back of people's

minds is global warming, overpopulation, terrorism etc. We don't know what is going to happen next, and how long the uncertainty is going to last. This uncertainty has many profound social psychological effects that may change consumer behavior completely. Although 'uncertain times' sounds negative, there is more good news in this trend than one might think.

### SAMPLES OF QUESTIONS THAT WILL BE ANSWERED

- *How do people react to uncertain times (short and long term)?*

- *How to survive uncertain times? What chances are there?*

- *What happens to the luxury and green markets in uncertain times?*

## VISUAL CULTURE

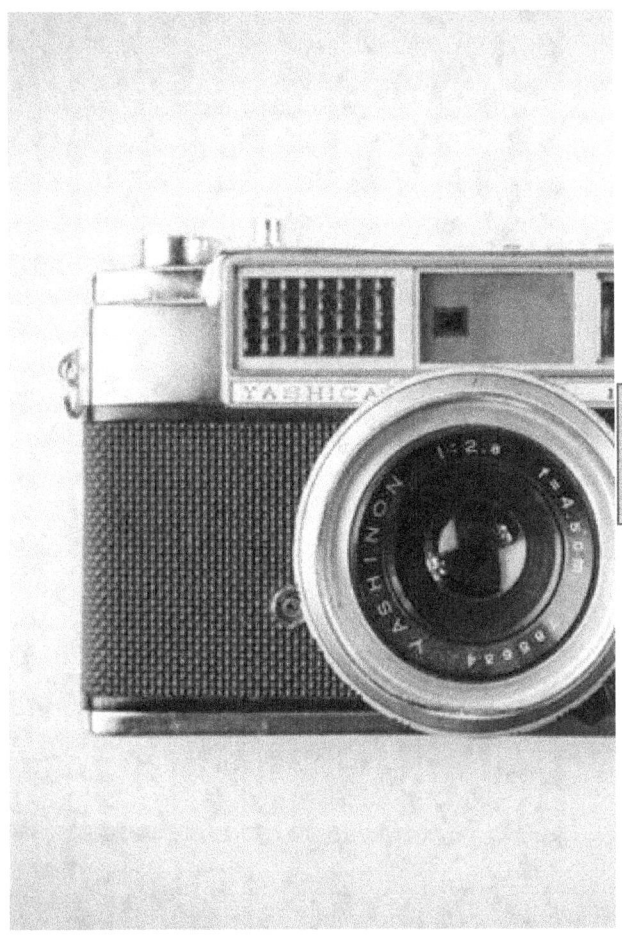

SAMPLES OF QUESTIONS THAT WILL
BE ANSWERED

- *What does the new visual culture look like?*
- *How can I use it in my marketing communication?*
- *What are the drivers and the effects of this visual culture?*

## CONNECTED SOCIETY

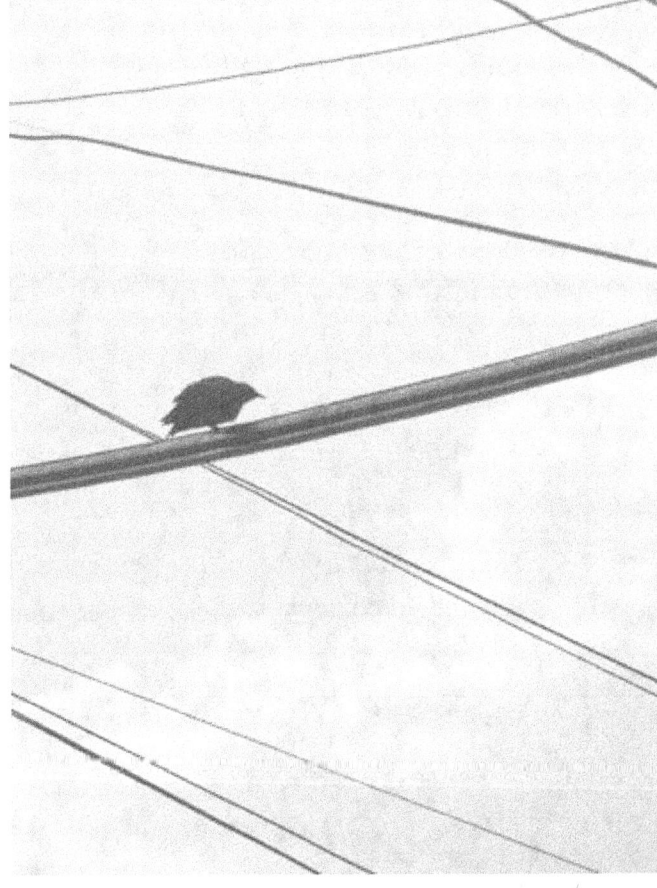

We are in the middle of the rise of a new visual culture, created by a young 'visual' generation. This generation grew up surrounded by a total abundance of images. Psychological research shows the result: this generation thinks visually and learns in images. Their way of working with images also differs from older generations. This new visual culture is often described in words, but rarely shown. This trend will show you how this visual culture is created and what it looks like. This trend also highlights the social cultural structures behind this new visual culture.

The digitalization that has taken place over the past fifteen years has fundamentally changed society. Everything and everybody is – to a certain degree – connected. This has changed not only our behaviour, but also the fundamentals of virtually every organization. This trend is about people connecting with each other, with products (and services) and with organizations.

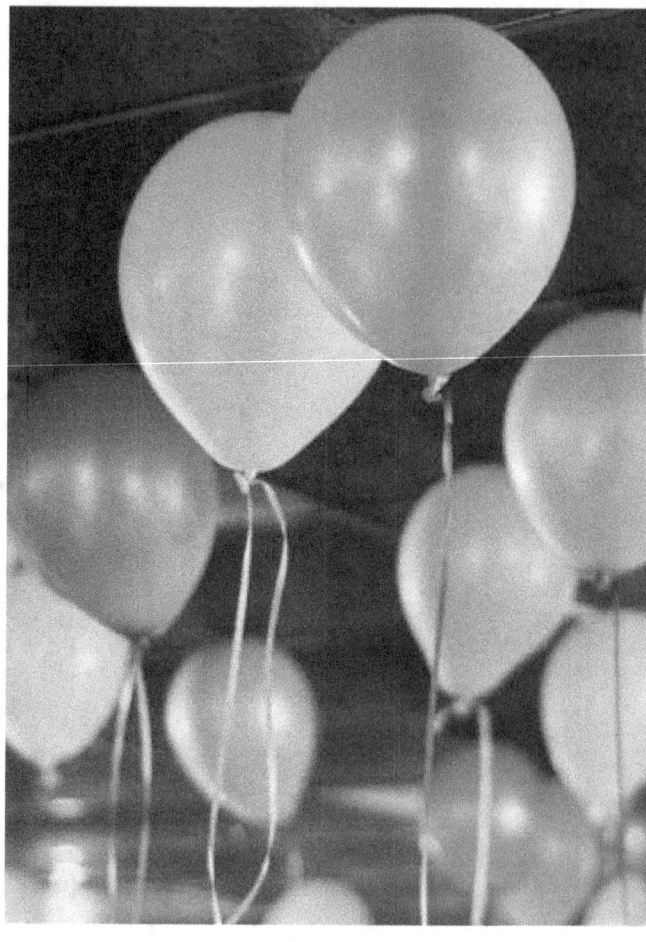

SAMPLES OF QUESTIONS THAT WILL BE ANSWERED

- *What are the sociocultural implications of new technology?*

- *What are the drivers behind recent technology trends?*

- *How can a brand serve the new, connected consumer?*

HEALTH TO HAPPINESS

This trend comprises all the latest on our physical and mental wellbeing in the 2010's. Health, wellness and happiness are converging into total wellbeing. People in the western industrialized world are demanding quality of life and a healthy work-life balance. People are trying to slow down their lives in a world where most things are going faster than ever.

SAMPLES OF QUESTIONS THAT WILL BE ANSWERED

- *How are health, wellness and happiness converging and why is this important for my organization?*
- *How do I keep my clients/employees happy?*
- *What are the differences among generations and sexes in terms of health, wellness and happiness?*

Games and playfulness are everywhere around us. They have an increasing impact on education, business and society in general. Technological advances such as mobile phones (i.e. compact game devices) and intuitive control have broadened and increased the gaming crowd. Everyone likes to play and the reasons why are quickly becoming clear. Game principles have proven to be highly motivating – and sometimes even addictive. The use of these game mechanisms can completely and positively change the way you(r business) work(s).

## POWER OF PLAY

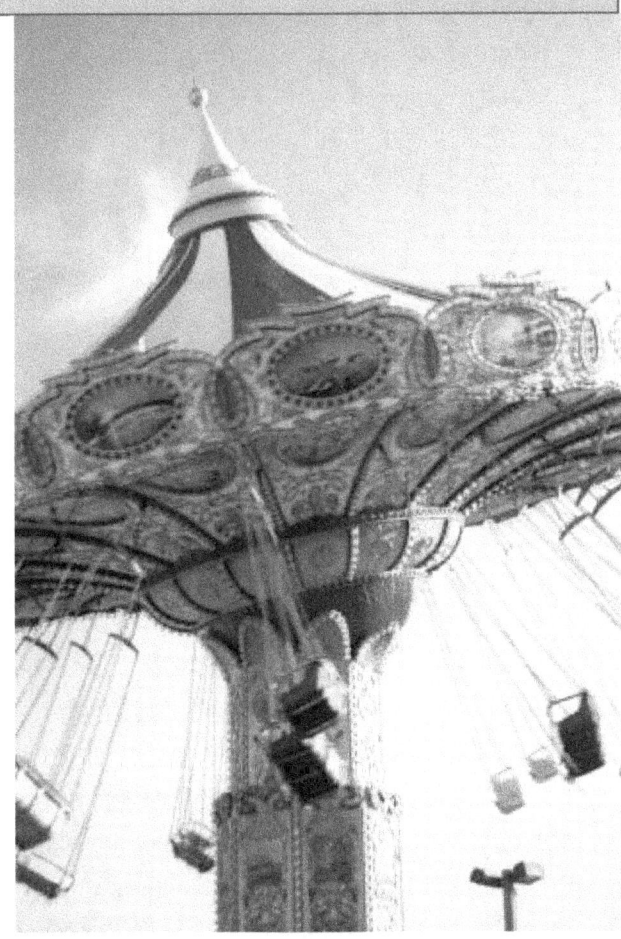

## SAMPLES OF QUESTIONS THAT WILL BE ANSWERED

- *How can you use play and game principles to increase your sales, motivate your students or engage your audience?*

-

- *In what way do different target groups (men / women / generations) differ in play?*

- *Will play be the future?*

## ABUNDANCE

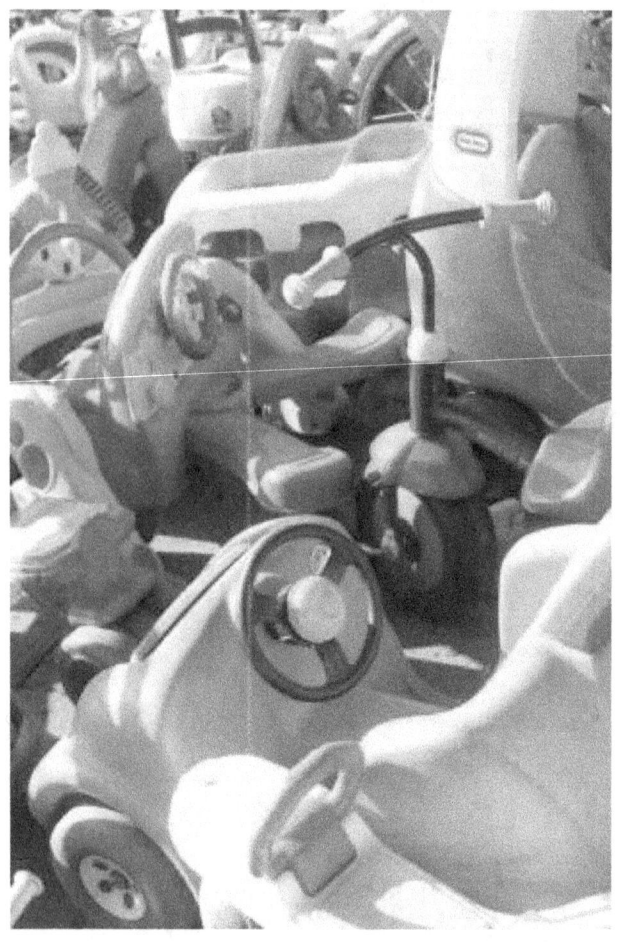

SAMPLES OF QUESTIONS THAT WILL
BE ANSWERED

- *How does abundance influence consumers' behavior?*

- *What can one help consumers in this time of abundance?*

- *How to reach consumers in world with abundant choice and abundant marketing?*

'The more the better' has been the mantra for a long time, but things have changed. The industrial revolution, mass production and the internet all have contributed to a growing amount of both 'things' and 'information'. We've entered the era of abundance, i.e. a more than adequate quantity or supply. Research shows there is an ideal number of choices, which is far lower than one might expect. Consumers feel overwhelmed and need filters in this abundant world. This trend explores the latest (and future) manifestations of abundance and the filter mechanisms which consumers use to make choices.

# 6 TIPS FOR SELLING YOUR HOME FAST

Claudia Stephens is the costume designer for La Discreta Enamorada and an associate professor in the Division of Theatre at SMU. For this production of Lope de Vega's play, she has based her designs on those of the 20th-century Spanish fashion designer, Cristobal Balenciaga: this is because the SMU

production of

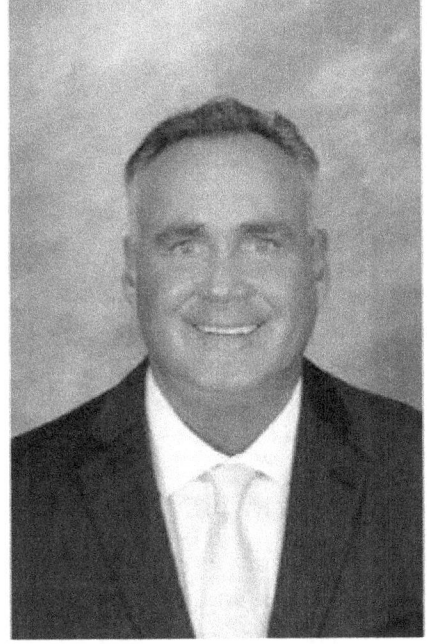

Your Real Estate Agent Todd Dowgialo

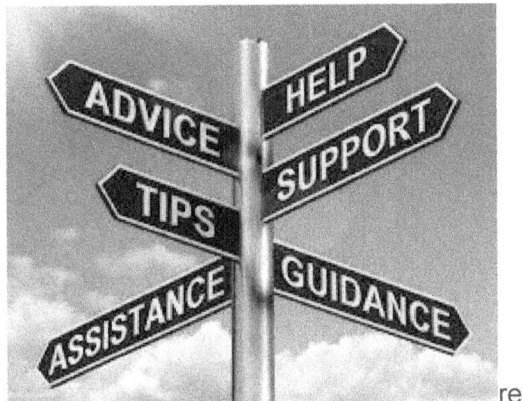

real estate images" />

Claudia Stephens is the costume designer for La Discreta Enamorada and an associate professor in the Division of Theatre at SMU.

31

For this production of Lope de Vega's play, she has based her designs on those of the 20th-century Spanish fashion designer, Cristobal Balenciaga: this is because the SMU production of In a down market, buyers are looking for a deal, so do your best to make them feel they're getting one.

Another tip is to offer a transferable home warranty, which can cost $300 to $400 for a one-year policy and will cover appliances, such as air conditioners and refrigerators, that fail. Depending on the policy, other appliances and house gadgets may be covered as well. A potential buyer may feel more at ease knowing that he or she will be covered against such problems, which could make your home more attractive than a competing home.

Finally, it's important to note that some buyers are motivated by the option to close in a short amount of time. If it is possible for you to close on the home within 30 to 60 days, this may set your deal apart and get you a contract.

Improve Curb Appeal
Sellers often overlook the importance of their home's curb appeal. The first thing a buyer sees is a home's external appearance and the way it fits into the surrounding neighborhood. Try to make certain that the exterior has a fresh coat of paint, and that the

bushes and lawn are well manicured. In real estate, appearances mean a lot. What better way to set your home apart than to make it attractive at first glance?

Get Your Home in "Move In" Condition
Aesthetics are important, but it's also important that doors, appliances and electrical and plumbing fixtures be in compliance with current building codes and in working order. Again, the idea is to have the home in move in condition and to give potential buyers the impression that they will be able to move right in and start enjoying their new home, rather than spending time and money fixing it up.

Pricing It Right
Regardless of how well you renovate and stage your home, it is still important to price the home appropriately. Consult a local real estate agent, read the newspapers and go to online real estate sites to see what comparable homes are going for in your area.

It's not always imperative to be the lowest priced home on the block, particularly when aesthetic and other significant improvements have been made. However, it is important that the listing price is not out of line with other comparable homes in the market. Try to put yourself in the buyer's shoes and then determine what a fair price might be. Have friends, neighbors and real

estate professionals tour the home and weigh in as well.

The Bottom Line
Selling a home in a down market requires a little extra work. Do everything you can to get the home in excellent shape and be prepared to make some small concessions at closing. These tips, coupled with an attractive price, will increase the odds of getting your home sold.

Mortgage Rates Take Huge Dip – 2.67% APR Rates now at 2.67% APR with no points – $225K mortgage for $904/mo. Process is easy & quotes are free! (2.67% APR 5/1 ARM). Calculate new payment now..

# Travel and Life Style

# Travel and life style

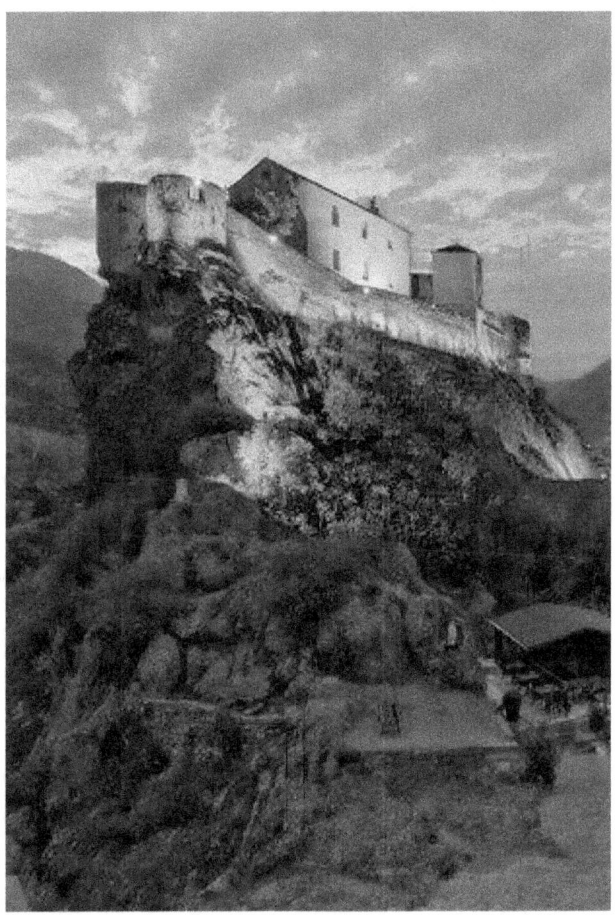

# CORSICA

**Napoleon's Soulful Island Home**

Two hundred years after Napoleon Bonaparte suffered his final military defeat, Corsica, his birthplace, stubbornly resists its own cultural Waterloo. Though this Mediterranean island has deep, historic ties to Italy and has been part of France since 1769, its 300,000 inhabitants retain a fierce pride in their own unique culture, including the proverb-rich Corsican tongue. But to keep that birthright vibrant in the face of tourism and its homogenizing effects, their battle remains constant.

Fortunately, most of the island's three million annual visitors come for the undeniable pleasures of the coast or for the thrill of visiting historic La Maison Bonaparte, in the city of Ajaccio. All of which leaves the island's mountainous interior largely untouched. "Go inland and you will find the soul of Corsica," advises Jean-Sébastien Orsini, director of a traditional Corsican polyphonic choir in the foothill town of Calanzana.

Olive groves and quiet villages dot the slopes and isolated valleys of the interior, vast swaths of which are protected by the Parc Naturel Régionale de Corse, which covers more than 40 percent of the island. Hiking trails lace forests of oak and pine. In the villages here, you encounter Corsicans who still feel passionately the adage "*Una lingua si cheta, un populu si more*—A language is silenced, a people die." *—Christopher Hall, @HallWriter*

**Travel Tips**

**When to Go:** May-June and September-October for walking, hiking, biking, and horseback riding; July-August (peak tourist season) for beaches and water sports

**How to Get Around:** Corsica has four commercial airports: Bastia (northeast), Ajaccio (southwest), Calvi (northwest), and Figari (south). Although driving is the most convenient way to travel around the island, many roads are narrow and winding. For shorter trips, hike, bike, or walk. Classic Journeys offers a six-night, seven-day Sardinia-Corsica cultural walking tour, and Corsican Places leads guided, weeklong cycling trips, including bike rental. Sign on with Tour Adventure to trek interior Corsica's bucket list-worthy GR20, a challenging 112-mile hiking route.

**Where to Stay:** Carpe Diem Palazzu, a six-suite, pastoral estate in the village of Eccica-Suarella, is a convenient base for both sea and mountain activities. Access to the Ajaccio airport, beaches, and water sports (including sailing, scuba diving, and jet skiing) is about 20 minutes away by car. Hotel staff can also arrange various inland adventures, such as horseback riding, canyoning, river kayaking, and fishing. To stay in the mountains, pitch a tent or rent a rustic cabin at Alivetu campground in Corte. Open May-September.

**Where to Eat or Drink:** *Castagne* (chestnut) is the flavor of Corsica. Look for chestnut-flavored ice cream, Pietra ale brewed from chestnut flour, *suppa di castagne* (chestnut soup), and chestnut-flour beignets stuffed with *brocciu*, Corsica's ricotta-like cheese (made with goat or ewe's milk).

**What to Buy:** Look for homegrown products such as fig jam, Muscat wine, and honey at the farmers market on Boulevard du Roi Jérôme in Ajaccio (closed Mondays). Pottery, stoneware, baskets, and knives are some of Corsica's best known artisanal items. Visit metalworker and cutlery maker Patrick Martin's*atelier* (workshop) in Calvi to see how Corsican knives and daggers are crafted and to buy a traditional shepherd's knife with a curved ram's horn handle.

**Practical Tip:** Bonifacio is touristy but worth a visit for the spectacular views. Walk the cliff-top path out toward Capo Pertusato just before dawn to see the cliffs change from chalky white to warm orange as the sun rises.

**What to Read Before You Go: Jérôme** Ferrari's philosophical Corsican epic*The Sermon on the Fall of Rome* (MacLehose Press, English edition, 2014), 2012 winner of France's top literary prize, follows a young philosophy student whose idealistic dreams are dashed by violence and corruption.

**Helpful Links:** Visit-Corsica and France Tourism

**Fun Fact:** The likelihood of spotting one of Corsica's European mouflon (wild sheep) is greater if you hike in the mountains, but the odds still aren't very good. The wild and wily sheep with outsize, sickle-shaped horns (males only) are nocturnal and live in the island's thickly wooded and rugged interior.

**Insider Tip From Christopher Hall:** In bakeries across the island, look for golden brown fiadone, a classic Corsican cheesecake of lemon zest and ricotta-like brocciu cheese made with sheep's or goat's milk.

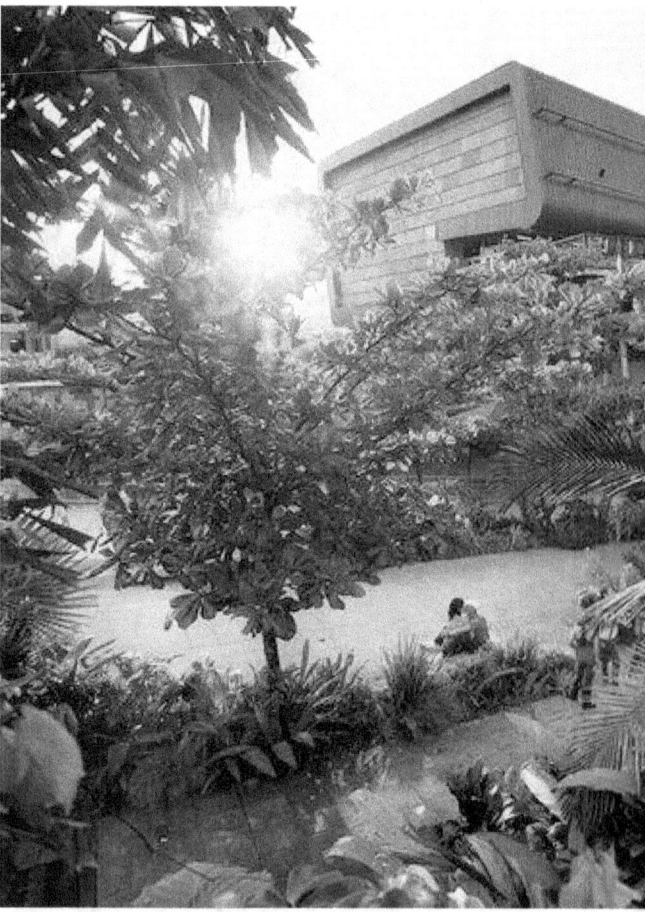

# MEDELLÍN, COLOMBIA

*Photograph by Heiko Meyer, laif/Redux*

## Famous for Flowers. Yes, Flowers.

Call it the Medellín miracle. Colombia's second city still has its vices, but the world's former cocaine capital has been rehabbed. Terrorism has ceded to tourism, thanks to visionary social policies that have transformed the once menacing city into a model metropolis. Slums where police feared to tread are now linked to the innovative business and cultural hub by the well-policed MetroCable, whisking visitors aloft to Barrio Santo Domingo, a new tourist hot spot where the black cubist España library perches dramatically over the shanties. Downtown, in the valley below, sunlight glints on skyscrapers and avant-garde architecture framed by Andean mountains—proof that a jewel is made complete by a stunning setting.

Art-filled public parks lie at the heart of the city's holistic makeover. Voluptuous sculptures by Medellín native Fernando Botero stud Plaza Botero, where the Museo de Antioquia displays paintings by Botero and Picasso. Nearby, office workers strolling Plaza de los Pies Descalzos ("barefoot park") cast off shoes and socks to rejuvenate amid a sensory Zen garden. Families flock to Parque Explora, with its interactive science exhibits and world-class aquarium. Self-assured young people in designer jeans swell Parque de Lleras, the city's epicenter for chic nightlife. Art-mad Medellinenses have even morphed a former steel mill into the Museo de Arte Moderno. Its Bonuar restaurant

serves Creole fusion fare spiced with live American-style blues.

Tradition? Relax. It scents the air when the City of Eternal Spring bursts into mid-summer bloom for the annual Feria de las Flores in August. The 58-year-old flower festival fills the streets with kaleidoscopic color, a winsome testament to Medellín's metamorphosis. —*Christopher P. Baker*

**Travel Tips**

**When to Go:** Year-round, average temperature remains about 72ºF every day; December-February is the dry season; May and October are the rainiest months; early August, Feria de las Flores (Flower Festival), a ten-day celebration of regional Antioquian culture; December, elaborate holiday light displays

**How to Get Around:** Use the modern Metro system to travel around the city for about a dollar per ride. For the best aerial views of Medellín, ride the Metrocables (cable cars) up the eastern slopes of the Aburra Valley (and over some of the city's poorest, mountainside favelas). Transfer (for about two dollars each way) to the scenic Metrocable line that extends up to the Parque Arvi nature preserve.

**Where to Stay:** The six-story Art Hotel Medellin in the upscale El Poblado neighborhood has an industrial loft vibe: brick walls, polished concrete floors, and exposed steel and wood beams. Rooms facing the atrium can seem cavelike, so book a brighter Superior or Executive room with a window overlooking the street. Walk a block to Parque Lleras, Medellín's popular restaurant and nightlife district.

**Where to Eat or Drink:** Two go-to Antioquian staples to try are *mondongo*—slow-simmered tripe and vegetable stew topped with a savory tomato and onion*criollo* sauce—and *bandeja paisa*, a platter piled high with filling foods like beans and rice, ground beef, avocado, plantain, and *chicharrón* (fried pork belly) and topped with a fried egg. The aptly named Mondongos serves both dishes at two Medellín locations.

**What to Buy:** Medellín's supersize malls are worth a visit for people-watching alone. At Poblado's posh El Tesoro Parque Comercial, fashion-forward Paisas (Medellín residents) stroll, dine, hang out on the atrium's cozy couches, and shop at upscale retail stores, including Arturo Calle and Tennis. The four-story, open-air mall also has a movie theater and a pint-size amusement park with a Ferris wheel and train.

**Cultural Tip:** Only tourists wear flip-flops, and local men are rarely spotted wearing shorts. To look more like a Paisa, leave the beachwear at home. Pack long pants and jeans instead.

**What to Read Before You Go:** Medellín native Héctor Abad's memoir *Oblivion* (Farrar, Straus and Giroux, reprint edition, 2013) is a profoundly moving tribute to his father, who was murdered by Colombian paramilitaries in 1987.

**Helpful Links:** Medellín Convention and Visitors Bureau and Medellín Living

**Fun Fact:** From Medellín, it's about a two-and-a-half-hour bus ride east to La Piedra del Peñol, or El Peñol (the Stone), a 721-foot monolith towering over the Embalse del Peñol hydroelectric dam. A switchback concrete staircase (built into a vertical crevice) leads up 649 steps to the top of the rock. Make the extra climb up the three-story observation tower for panoramic views of the islands and man-made lakes below.

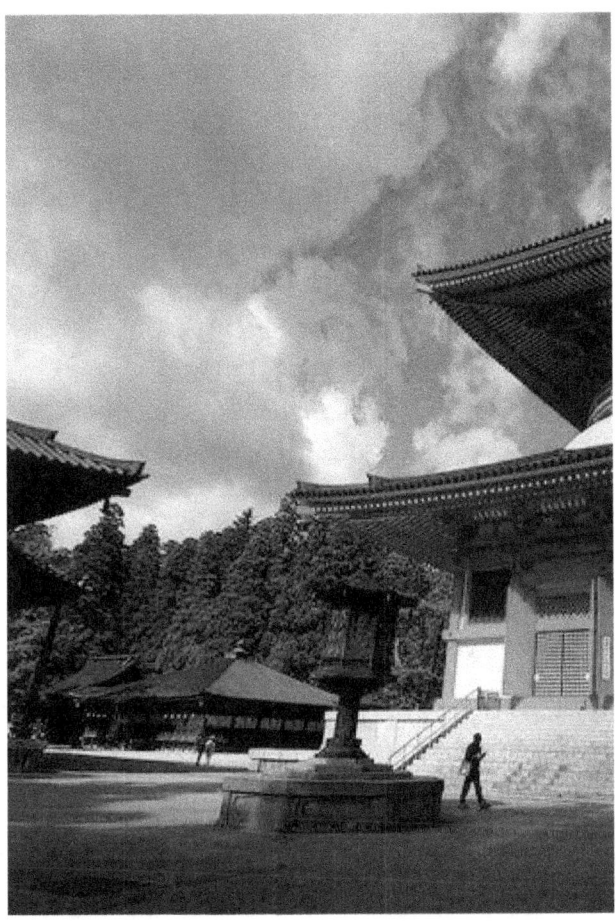

# KOYASAN, JAPAN

*Photograph by Jeremy Horner, Panos Pictures*

**Let There Be Enlightenment**

The austere heart of Japanese Buddhism beats loudly at Koyasan, a monastic complex that lies two hours by train south of Osaka. Koyasan marks its 1,200th anniversary in 2015.

Established by revered scholar-monk Kobo Daishi in 816 as the headquarters for his Shingon school of Esoteric Buddhism, Koyasan remains one of Japan's most pristine and sacred sites,

37

manifesting a masculine side of Japan worlds away from the hostesses and Hello Kittys of Kyoto.

"Koyasan is purity," says a monk after a crack-of-dawn fire ceremony, where a priest burns wooden wish-tablets to the boom of a *taiko* drum and the sprinkling of herbs and oils on high-leaping flames. Staying in one of the temples that welcome guests here opens a portal onto everyday monastic life. Waking to enshrouding mists, visitors are invited to join morning chants swirled by cymbals, gongs, and incense. At night, no-nonsense monks who began the day hand-scrubbing wooden hallways roughly plop vegetarian feasts in front of visitors.

Kobo Daishi is believed to live here still, sitting in eternal meditation in an elaborate mausoleum, and through the centuries, Japan's most rich and powerful have built palatial sepulchers here as well. At night, a ghostly lantern-lit trail winds among the moss-covered stones deep into the mystery and majesty of ancient Japan. *—Don George, @don_george*

**Travel Tips**

**When to Go:** Weekdays (April-November) to avoid weekend tourist crowds; June 15, Aoba Festival's colorful float procession and drumming; August 13-16, Mandokuyo-e (Candle Festival).

**How to Get Around:** At Osaka's Namba Station, purchase Nankai Electric Railway's Koyasan World Heritage Ticket, which includes round-trip transportation (train, cable car, and bus) and discount coupons for admission tickets and stores. Take the Koya Line to the last stop, Gokurakubashi Station(about 90 minutes). The Koyasan cable car boarding area is inside the station. From here it's a steep, five-minute cable car ride up to Koyasan Eki-mae Station and the Nankai Rinkan bus terminal. Board the tourist bus to stop at all major Koyasan sites, including the Koyasan Tourist Association office, where you can pick up a map.

**Where to Stay:** Fifty-two of Koyasan's temples offer guest accommodations, called shukubo. Rates, comfort levels, and amenities vary from dormlike to spa-retreat minimalism. Breakfast and dinner are typically included. Get up at dawn to observe the monks' devotional morning chants and fire ceremonies. Make reservations via the official Shukubo Koyasan website, or book directly with temples such as Fukuchi-in, Eko-in, and Kumagai-ji, which have English-language websites.

**What to Eat or Drink:** Shukubo guests are treated to *shojin-ryori* (devotion cuisine), the strictly vegan and subtly flavored (no garlic or onion) fare of Japanese Buddhist monks. The multicourse Koyasan shojin-ryori dinner—typically served in tiny lacquer bowls either on trays in your room or in a separate dining room—often includes sticky *goma-dofu* (sesame tofu), plus rice, tea, and dishes such as *koya-dofu* (freeze-dried tofu), vegetable tempura, and *sashimi konnyaku* (thin slices of a gelatinous core made from the yamlike konjac root).

**What to Buy:** Visit Juzuya Shirobe (a World Heritage Ticket discount-coupon partnering store) to shop for Shingon-style Buddhist *juzu* prayer beads and bracelets, small *jisuzu* bells, incense, and other Buddhist devotional items.

**Cultural Tip:** For an English-language Koyasan tour, rent a Koyasan Audio Guide from the Koyasan Shukubo Association, or book a two- or four-hour walking tour or custom trek with the Koyasan Interpreter Guide Club.

**What to Read Before You Go:** Anthropologist, writer, and filmmaker Christal Whelan's *Kansai Cool: A Journey Into the Cultural Heartland of Japan* (Tuttle Publishing, 2014) includes a chapter devoted to the Koyasan Buddhist monastery.

**Helpful Links:** <u>Koyasan Shukubo Association</u>, <u>Koyasan Shingon Buddhism</u>,<u>Koyasan Cross-Cultural Communication Network</u>, and <u>Koyasan Tourist Association</u>

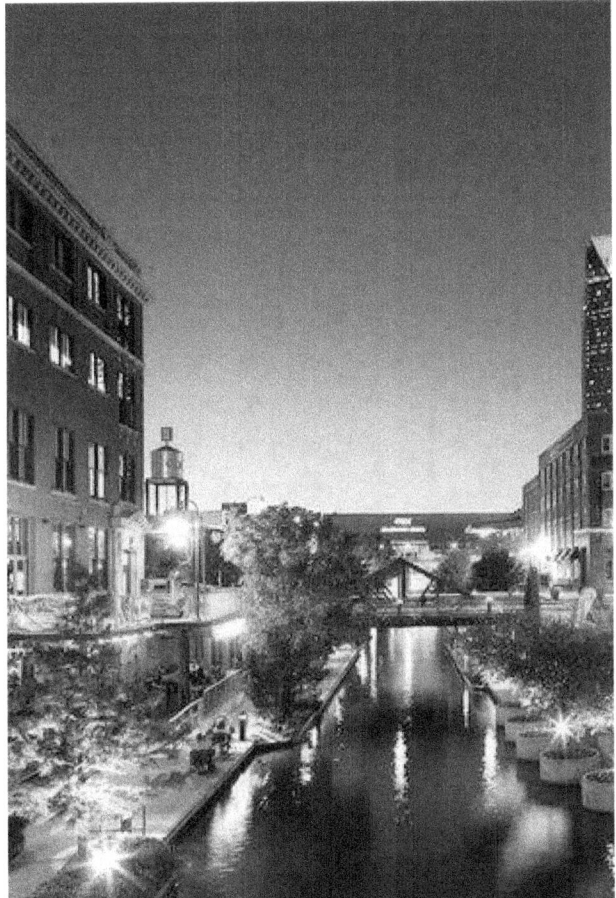

# OKLAHOMA CITY, OKLAHOMA

*Photograph by Walter Bibikow, Getty*

**Pride of the Plains**

Oklahoma City has never been "mighty pretty," despite the shout-out from Bobby Troup's iconic "Route 66." To look at, it's been more like the beer-gut metropolis spilling across the Great Plains. But things have changed.

The central Oklahoma River has a community boathouse and a new West River Trail. An 11-acre white-water rafting center is due in 2015. Local architect firms and coffee roasters that wouldn't be out of place in *Portlandia* now line once dormant Automobile Alley. And then there's MidTown. Not long ago a den of crackhouses and abandoned lots just north of downtown's 1995 bombing site, MidTown has sprouted condos, a boutique hotel, and Dust Bowl Lanes, a Tulsan import, with its 1970s-style bowling alley. The city even plans to add a streetcar loop downtown in 2017.

This is Oklahoma?

"We're such a blank canvas that even people *from Austin* are moving here," says Hunter Wheat, who launched MidTown's Blue Garten last year, a one-block food truck complex with open-air movies and live bands. "I'm just happy to see it's growing into the city I always knew it could be." —*Robert Reid,* <u>*@reidontravel*</u>

**Travel Tips**

**When to Go:** April 26, <u>Oklahoma City Memorial Marathon, Half Marathon, and 5K</u>, which supports the <u>Oklahoma City</u>

National Memorial and Museum; June 10-14, deadCENTER Film Festival; October 2-5, Oklahoma Regatta Festival.

**How to Get Around:** From Will Rogers World Airport, rent a car or take the shuttle bus for the 15-minute ride downtown or to Bricktown, the city's entertainment district. Amtrak's Heartland Flyer also runs daily between Fort Worth, Texas, and Bricktown's Sante Fe Depot. Downtown, walk or use Spokies, Oklahoma City's bike-share program. Daily memberships are $5 and include unlimited 30-minute rides. For longer explorations, ride the Oklahoma City EMBARK public buses or rent a bike at Schlegel Bicycles in the Automobile Alley district.

**Where to Stay:** Housed in OKC's first skyscraper (built in 1910) and restored to its original grandeur in 2006, the luxurious 12-story Colcord Hotel combines convenience (free downtown shuttle service) with pampering (complimentary coffee or tea wake-up calls delivered to your room). The Colcord is within walking distance of the Myriad Botanical Gardens, the Oklahoma City National Memorial and Museum,

and Chesapeake Energy Arena, home to the NBA's Oklahoma City Thunder.

**Where to Eat or Drink:** Join the local "Que-heads" at Back Door BBQ, where the daily Beast-wich (such as pulled pork piled high and topped with mustard, mayo, spring mix, sweet pickle relish, red peppers, and red onions) could be enough to cover both lunch and dinner. Or follow the aroma of smoky pecan wood to theWedge Deep Deuce Pizzeria, where handcrafted pies such as the **Truffle-Shuffle (*truffle oil, sage, cremini mushrooms, spinach, roasted chicken, parmesan, and mozzarella*)** are baked bubbly and golden brown in a wood-fired oven.

**What to Buy:** Support Keep It Local OK's locally owned and operated shops, such as hip and playful Plenty Mercantile in the historic Automobile Alley district. Located in a building that housed a 1920s Chevrolet dealership, Plenty specializes in consciously produced home goods, foods, and gifts, including Oklahoma-made Strong Tonic, Kize Bars, and Always Greener turf doormats. There's also a rooftop event space, where Plenty regularly hosts community workshops, gardening classes, wine tastings, intimate dinners, and brunch.

**What to Read Before You Go:** The hero of master storyteller Elmore Leonard's 40th novel *The Hot Kid* (HarperTorch, reprint edition, 2006) is a quick-draw U.S. marshal in Depression-era Oklahoma.

**Helpful Links:** Oklahoma City Tourism and Oklahoma Tourism and Recreation

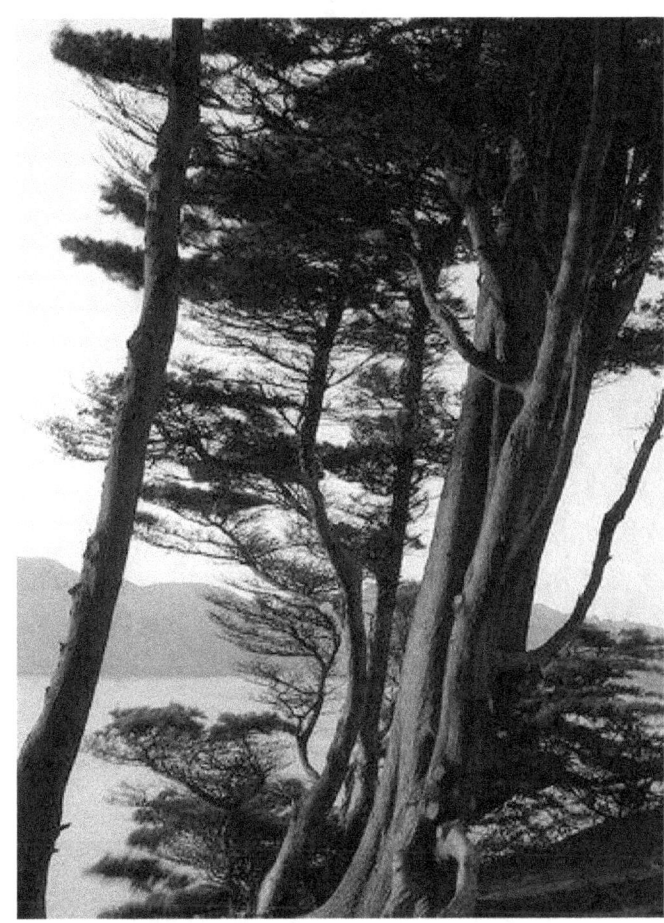

# THE PRESIDIO, SAN FRANCISCO

*Photograph by Ron Niebrugge, Mira Images*

**From Spanish Conquistadores to** *Star Wars*

If the San Francisco Peninsula resembles a forearm ending in a fist, then the Presidio is the topmost

**Fun Fact:** It only took a day for Oklahoma City to become a city. The day was April 22, 1889, when the federal government held the first "land run" into the Unassigned Lands (territory not designated for a specific Indian nation) of modern-day western Oklahoma. More than 10,000 men, women, and children moved to Oklahoma City that day, founding the city that would become the state capital in 1910.

knuckle-by-the-Bay. The virile park of viridian woods and knockout vistas can make travelers forget its original function was for war, not Instagram. To San Franciscans, it's both muse and playground—with the latest addition being the newly reopened Officers' Club, reimagined as a local hub for exhibits, performances, and dining.

Established by Spanish conquistadores in 1776, the military garrison of Saint Francis and its 2.3 square miles defended the bay from any invaders tempted by the riches of Alta California. For the next 218 years, soldiers stood guard against the machinations of empires. But the English, Russian, Japanese, and Klingons—*Star Trek*'s Starfleet Command is headquartered here—never came. The base became a coveted U.S. Army assignment. Officers dream of three things, the saying went: "to make colonel, to die and go to heaven, and to be posted to the Presidio."

In 1994, ownership passed from the Army to the National Park Service. Now the Presidio is a self-sustaining trust, thanks to rents paid by one-percenters like George Lucas, whose Lucasfilms office here blessed with a Yoda sculpture on a fountain. (Critics prefer sculptor Andy Goldsworthy's nearly hundred-foot-tall "Spire," near the Arguello Gate.) But why nitpick? Instead, savor a hot chocolate after a hike on Crissy Field. Listen for the whiz-whir generated by bikers pumping down

Lincoln Boulevard above North Baker Beach's clothing-optional sunbathers. Delight in the eucalyptus-scented footpath called Lovers Lane. The Presidio, young Skywalker! The Force is strong with this one. *—Andrew Nelson,@andrewnelson*

Travel Tips

**When to Go:** April, May, October, and November typically are the best months to visit due to the warm, sunny weather and minimal fog (providing better views of the Golden Gate Bridge). Weekdays are less crowded.

**How to Get Around:** From San Francisco International Airport rent a car, or ride BART (Bay Area Rapid Transit) to the Embarcadero station. From here (at the corner of Drumm and Market Streets), take the free Presidio shuttle bus (9:30 a.m. to 4 p.m. on weekdays and 10:30 a.m. to 7:30 p.m on weekends).

**Where to Stay:** Built in 1903, the gracious Georgian Revival-style Pershing Hall (formerly used to house unmarried and visiting U.S. Army officers) was restored in 2011 and reopened in April 2012 as the Inn at the Presidio. The main inn includes five guest rooms and 17 suites replicating the layout of the original officers' quarters. The adjacent, single-level Funston House (built in 1889 and opened to guests in 2013) has three guest rooms and one master suite. When the weather is clear, many of the third-floor main inn suites have Golden Gate Bridge views. Rates include a continental buffet breakfast and an evening wine and cheese reception (milk and cookies for younger guests).

**Where to Eat or Drink:** Housed in the former mess hall, The Commissary at the Presidio serves light breakfasts, eat-in and takeout lunches, and a full dinner menu (reservations recommended). Award-winning chef Traci Des Jardins mainly uses locally sourced ingredients to prepare the Spanish-influenced California cuisine (salt cod fritters, Marin Sun Farms burgers, and roasted chicken with Marcona almonds and dates). Most seating is communal. To watch the chefs prepare your meal, request a place at the bar surrounding the open kitchen.

**What to Buy:** At the Presidio, Warming Hut Bookstore and Café, located at the west end of Crissy Field; the Golden Gate Bridge Pavilion; and the Fort Point Bookstore have the best selection of Presidio-related souvenirs, gear, and books.

**Practical Tip:** To stay warm (and avoid looking like a tourist) wear long pants and several light layers if visiting the

Presidio in summer (June-August) when the weather is typically cold and foggy.

**What to Read Before You Go**: Set at the Presidio, *The Enlisted Men's Club*(Running Meter Press, 2014) is the first in a trilogy of military-life novels penned by late author and Vietnam War veteran Gary Reilly.

**Helpful Links:** Presidio of San Francisco and San Francisco Travel

**Fun Fact:** Following the attack on Pearl Harbor, the executive order authorizing the internment of Japanese Americans was issued at the Presidio. At the same time that their family members were being relocated to internment camps, Japanese-American linguist soldiers were training at the Presidio for critical military language duties such as translation and negotiation. The soldiers' training site, which reopened in 2013 as the Military Intelligence Service (MIS)Historic Learning Center, is open to the public Saturdays and Sundays, 12-5 p.m.

**2 BOOK AND MAGAZINE OFFERS ARE AVAILABLE FOR YOU.**

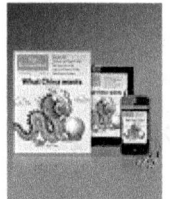 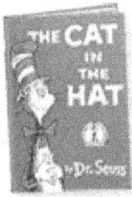

## 5 BOOKS FOR $5.95

*Official Dr. Seuss Book Club*

Hardcover Books - Free Shipping!

## FIRST 12 WEEKS FOR $15

*The Economist*

Insights not found anywhere else. Subscribe today.

# Free Printable Coupon

# Free Printable Coupon

# Free Printable Coupon

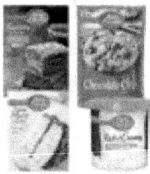

## SAVE 75¢ ON TWO

*Betty Crocker®*

when you buy TWO Betty Crocker® Ready to Spread Frosting, Supreme Brownie Mix, Dessert Bar Mix, SuperMoist® Cake Mix, OR Cookie

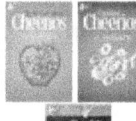

## SAVE $1.00 ON TWO

*Big G Cereals®*

when you buy any TWO BOXES Cheerios™ cereals listed: Frosted Cheerios™ • Apple Cinnamon Cheerios™ • Banana Nut Cheerios™...

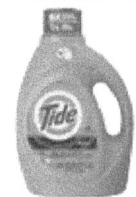

## $1.00 OFF

*TIDE®*

ONE Tide® Detergent 40 oz or larger (excludes Tide® Simply, Tide® PODS, 10 oz and trial/travel size)

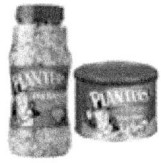

SAVE $1.00

## PLANTERS

on any TWO (2) PLANTERS Nuts or Peanut Butter (6 oz. or larger)

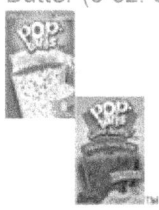

SAVE $1.00

## Kellogg's® Pop-Tarts®

on any THREE Kellogg's® Pop-Tarts® Toaster Pastries

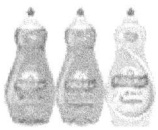

SAVE $0.35

## Palmolive®

On any Palmolive® Liquid Dish Soap (10 oz or larger)

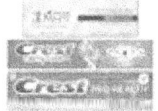

$1.50 OFF

## CREST®

45

TWO Crest® Toothpastes 3.0 oz or more or Liquid Gel (excludes Crest® Cavity, Baking Soda, Tartar Control and trial/travel size)

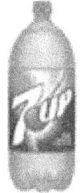

SAVE 55¢

## 7UP®

on ONE (1) 2-liter bottle of any flavor* 7UP® (Reg. or Diet)

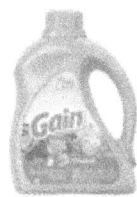

$1.00 OFF

## GAIN®

ONE Gain® Laundry Detergent 40 oz or larger liquid or 22 load or larger powder (excludes Fireworks and trial/travel size)

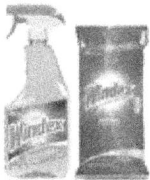

SAVE $1.00

## Windex®

on any ONE (1) Windex® product (excludes 4ct Electronics Wipes and trial/travel sizes)

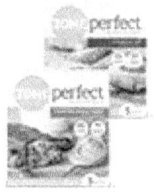

$2.00 OFF

*ZonePerfect®*

Any two (2) ZonePerfect® 5-count Multipacks

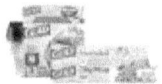

SAVE $1.00

*Glad®*

on any Glad® Food Protection Item

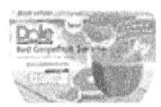

$0.75 OFF

*DOLE Fruit Bowls®*

ONE (1) PACKAGE OF DOLE RED GRAPEFRUIT SUNRISE

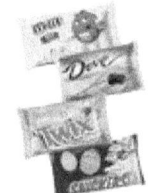

SAVE $1.00

*MARS Easter*

on any TWO (2) M&M'S® (2 oz.+), DOVE® Chocolate, MINIS MIX™, TWIX®, SNICKERS®,

MILKY WAY®, 3 MUSKETEERS® Brands (4.5 oz.+)

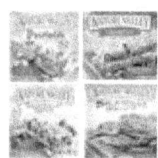

SAVE 50¢ ON TWO

*Nature Valley™*

when you buy TWO BOXES any Nature Valley™ Granola Bars (5 count or larger), Nature Valley™ Nut Crisp Bars, Nature Valley™ Gra...

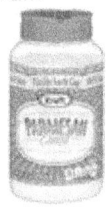

SAVE $1.50

*KRAFT*

on any ONE (1) KRAFT 100% Grated Parmesan Cheese, 16oz or larger

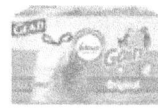

SAVE $1.00

*Glad®*

on any Glad® OdorShield® Trash Bag

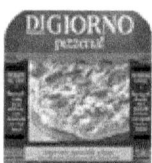

# My Connections Magazine

SAVE $2.00

## DIGIORNO®

when you buy any TWO (2) DIGIORNO® pizzeria!™ pizzas

$1.00 OFF

## CREST®

ONE Crest® 3D White Toothpaste 4.1 oz or larger (excludes trial/travel size)

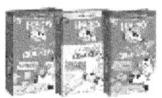

BUY 1 GET 1 FREE (UP TO $4.29)

## Horizon®

Any Horizon® Snack Crackers, Sandwich Crackers or Snack Grahams

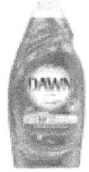

25¢ OFF

## DAWN®

ONE Dawn® product (excludes trial/travel size)

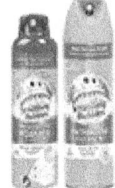

SAVE $1.00

## Scrubbing Bubbles®

on any ONE (1) Scrubbing Bubbles® Bath Cleaning product

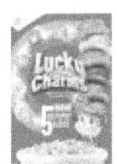

SAVE 50¢ ON ONE

## Big G Cereals®

when you buy ONE BOX Lucky Charms® cereal

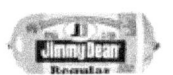

SAVE $1.00

## Jimmy Dean®

on any ONE (1) Jimmy Dean® Fresh Roll Sausage. Available at Walmart.

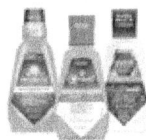

$1.10 OFF

## CREST®

ONE Crest® Rinse 473mL or larger (excludes trial/travel size)

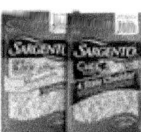

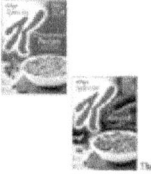
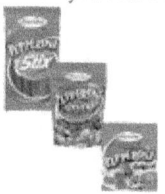
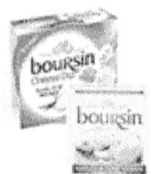
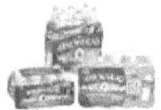
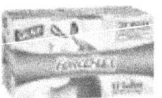
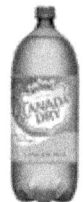
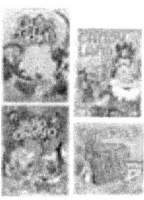

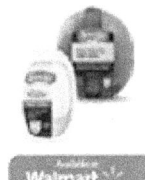

SAVE $1.00

*Sara Lee® Deli*

on 1 lb. of Sara Lee® Premium Meat at the service deli OR 1 package of Sara Lee® Pre-Sliced Meat located in the deli section

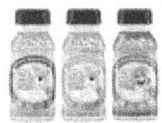

SAVE $3.00

*PediaSure®*

on any two (2) PediaSure® or PediaSure SideKicks® products

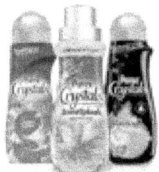

SAVE $3.00

*Purex® Crystals*

on any TWO (2) Purex® Crystals Fragrance Boosters

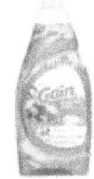

25¢ OFF

*GAIN®*

ONE Gain® Dishwashing Liquid (excludes 9oz and trial/travel size)

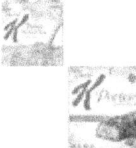

SAVE $2.00

*Kellogg's™ Special K™*

on any TWO Kellogg's™ Special K™ Protein Shakes and/or Meal Bars

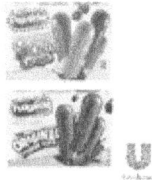

SAVE $1.00

*Popsicle®*

Off any Two (2) Popsicle® Products (9 count or higher)

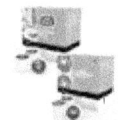

SAVE $1.00

*select K-Cup® pods*

Any ONE (1) box of Green Mountain Coffee® or The Original Donut Shop® K-Cup® pods

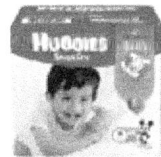

## SAVE $2.00
### HUGGIES®

on any ONE (1) package of HUGGIES® Diapers

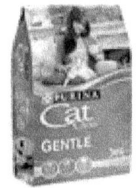

## SAVE $1.05
### Purina® Cat Chow®

on one (1) 3.15lb or larger bag of Purina® Cat Chow® brand dry cat food, any variety.

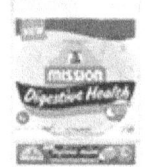

## SAVE $1.00
### Mission Tortillas

on One (1) Package of Mission Digestive Health Tortillas

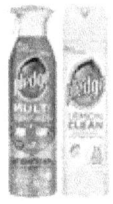

## SAVE $1.00
### Pledge®

on any ONE (1) Pledge® Furniture Care product

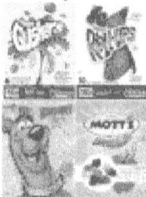

## SAVE 50¢ ON TWO
### Betty Crocker®

when you buy TWO BOXES any flavor/variety Betty Crocker® Fruit Shapes, Fruit by the Foot®, Fruit Gushers® or Fruit Roll-Ups®...

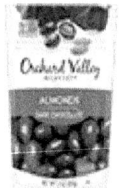

## $0.75 OFF
### Orchard Valley Harvest®

on TWO (2) Orchard Valley Harvest Grab & Go bags

# BABY AND TODDLER COUPONS

**21 BABY AND TODDLER OFFERS ARE AVAILABLE FOR YOU.**

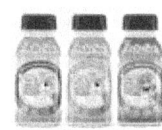

## SAVE $3.00
### PediaSure®

on any two (2) PediaSure® or PediaSure SideKicks® products

**$2.00 OFF**

*DREFT®*

ONE Dreft® Detergent (excludes trial/travel size)

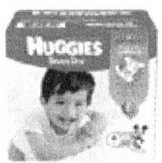

**SAVE $2.00**

*HUGGIES®*

on any ONE (1) package of HUGGIES® Diapers

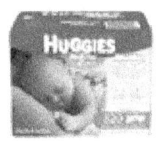

**SAVE $1.00**

*HUGGIES®*

on any ONE (1) package of HUGGIES® Wipes (180 ct. or larger)

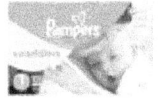

**$1.50 OFF**

*PAMPERS®*

ONE Pampers® Swaddlers Diapers (excludes trial/travel size)

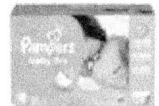

**$1.50 OFF**

*PAMPERS®*

ONE Pampers® Baby Dry Diapers (excludes trial/travel size)

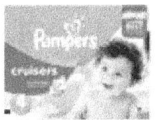

**$1.50 OFF**

*PAMPERS®*

ONE Pampers® Cruisers Diapers (excludes trial/travel size)

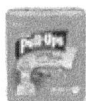

**SAVE $2.00**

*PULL-UPS®*

on any ONE (1) package of PULL-UPS® Training Pants (Jumbo Pack or larger)

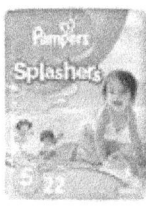

**$1.50 OFF**

*PAMPERS®*

ONE Pampers® Splashers Swim Pant (excludes trial/travel size)

SAVE $3.50

*PULL-UPS®*

on any TWO (2) packages of PULL-UPS®
Training Pants (Jumbo Pack or larger)

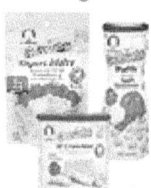

SAVE $1.00

*Gerber® Graduates®*

off any 3 Gerber® Graduates® Puffs, Lil'
Crunchies®, or Yogurt Melts™ items

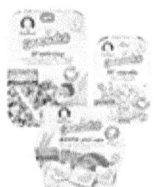

SAVE $1.00

*Gerber® Graduates®*

off any 3 Gerber® Graduates® Meals or Sides
items

SAVE $1.00

*NUK®*

Off Any (1) ONE NUK PACIFIER

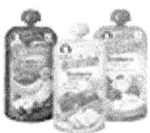

SAVE $1.00

*Gerber® Graduates®*

off any 4 Gerber® Graduates® Grabbers™
items

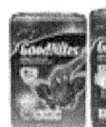
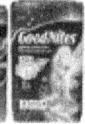

SAVE $2.00

*GOODNITES®*

on ONE package of GOODNITES® Product
(Underwear, Bed Mats, or GOODNITES* TRU-
FIT* Starter Pack or Refills) Jumbo Pack or
larger

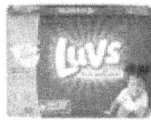

50¢ OFF

*LUVS®*

ONE Luvs® Diapers (excludes trial/travel size)

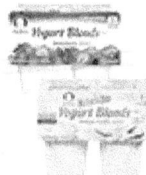

SAVE $1.00

*Gerber®*

off any 2 Gerber® or Graduates® Yogurt Blends items

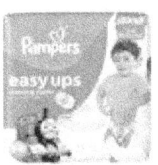

$1.50 OFF

*PAMPERS®*

ONE Pampers® Easy Ups Training Pants (excludes trial/travel size)

ALL OTHER COUPONS **(382)**

SAVE $3.00

*Boudreaux's*

on ONE (1) can of BOUDREAUX'S® RASH PREVENTOR™

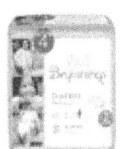

*Walgreens*

$1.50 OFF

*Well Beginnings*

ON ONE BAG OR BOX OF WELL BEGINNINGS DIAPERS (EXCLUDES 2CT TRIAL PACKS)

53

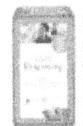 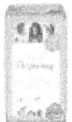

*Walgreens*

SAVE $1.50

*Well Beginnings*

one ONE (1) pack of WELL BEGINNINGS™ TRAINING PANTS (excluding trial packs)

ALL OTHER COUPONS **(382)**

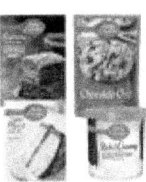

SAVE 75¢ ON TWO

*Betty Crocker®*

when you buy TWO Betty Crocker® Ready to Spread Frosting, Supreme Brownie Mix, Dessert Bar Mix, SuperMoist® Cake Mix, OR Cookie

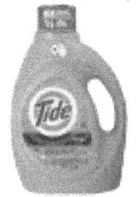

$1.00 OFF

*TIDE®*

ONE Tide® Detergent 40 oz or larger (excludes Tide® Simply, Tide® PODS, 10 oz and trial/travel size)

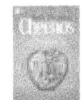

## SAVE $1.00 ON TWO

*Big G Cereals®*

when you buy any TWO BOXES Cheerios™ cereals listed: Frosted Cheerios™ • Apple Cinnamon Cheerios™ • Banana Nut Cheerios™...

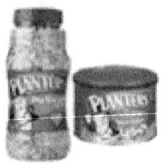

## SAVE $1.00

*PLANTERS*

on any TWO (2) PLANTERS Nuts or Peanut Butter (6 oz. or larger)

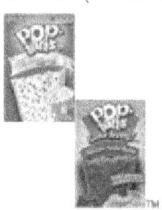

## SAVE $1.00

*Kellogg's® Pop-Tarts®*

on any THREE Kellogg's® Pop-Tarts® Toaster Pastries

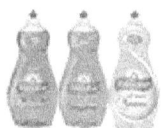

## SAVE $0.35

*Palmolive®*

On any Palmolive® Liquid Dish Soap (10 oz or larger)

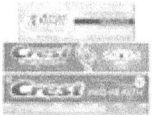

## $1.50 OFF

*CREST®*

TWO Crest® Toothpastes 3.0 oz or more or Liquid Gel (excludes Crest® Cavity, Baking Soda, Tartar Control and trial/travel size)

## HEALTH CARE COUPONS

**43 HEALTH CARE OFFERS ARE AVAILABLE FOR YOU.**

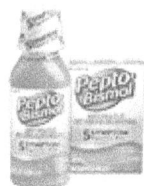

## 50¢ OFF

*PEPTO-BISMOL™*

ONE Pepto-Bismol™ product (excludes trial/travel size)

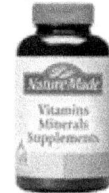

## $2.00 OFF

*Nature Made®*

on any Two (2) Nature Made® Products

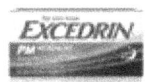

**SAVE $1.50**

*Excedrin®*

On any one (1) Excedrin® PM Headache 24 count

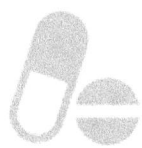

**UP TO 75% OFF!**

*FREE Prescription Discounts*

Free prescription savings at your pharmacy!

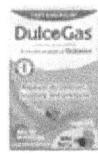

**SAVE $3.00**

*DulcoGas™*

On the purchase of ONE (1) DulcoGas™ 18 count or larger. Redeemable at Walgreens

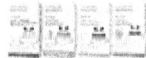

**SAVE $3.00**

*Zarbee's® Naturals*

On any (1) ONE Zarbee's® Naturals Baby Vitamins (Multivitamin, Probiotic, Omega 3 or Vitamin D)

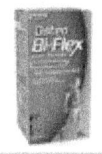

**SAVE $3.00**

*Osteo Bi-Flex®*

on any ONE (1) Osteo Bi-Flex® Joint Supplement (excluding edge) (Redeemable at Walmart)

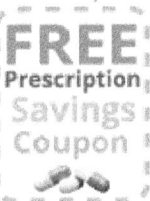

**UP TO 75% OFF!**

*FREE Prescription Discount*

Free prescription savings at your pharmacy!

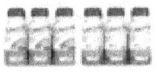

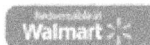

**SAVE $2.00**

*Glucerna®*

when you buy any ONE (1) Glucerna® Product

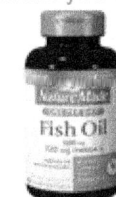

## $1.00 OFF

*Nature Made®*

Any One (1) Nature Made® Fish Oil (excludes 30 count)

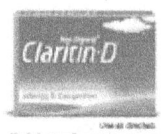

Sold at pharmacy or service counter
(no prescription needed in most states)

## SAVE $4.00

*Claritin-D®*

on any Non-Drowsy Claritin-D® Allergy Product (15ct or larger)

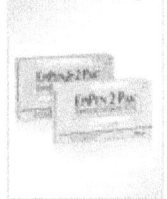

## $0 CO-PAY OFFER

*EpiPen® (epinephrine) Auto-Injector*

Are you eligible? Click for Terms and Conditions.

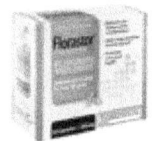

## CLICK AND SAVE $3

*Florastor®*

The daily probiotic for digestive health.

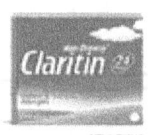

Get Claritin Clear.*

## SAVE $6.00

*Claritin*

on any Non-Drowsy Claritin® (45ct or larger)

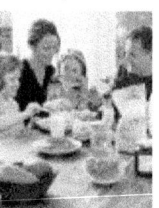

## ANAPHYLAXIS TREATMENT

*Money-Saving Offer*

Learn how to save on a prescription treatment.

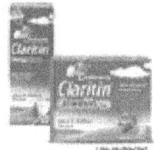

Get Claritin Clear.*

## SAVE $3.00

*Claritin®*

on any Non-Drowsy Children's Claritin® Chewables (20ct or larger)

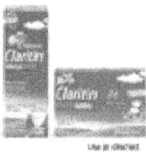

Get Claritin Clear.*

## SAVE $2.00

*Claritin®*

on any Non-Drowsy Children's Claritin® Syrup (4oz or larger) or RediTabs (10ct)

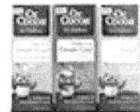

Jobs, Careers, personals, sale, buy, for rent, lease, and other oppourtunities.

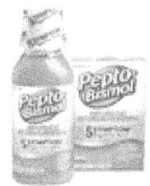
# Classifieds

Online at:

http://www.anaheimpublishing.co

Anaheim Publishing co.

Anywhere America classifieds.

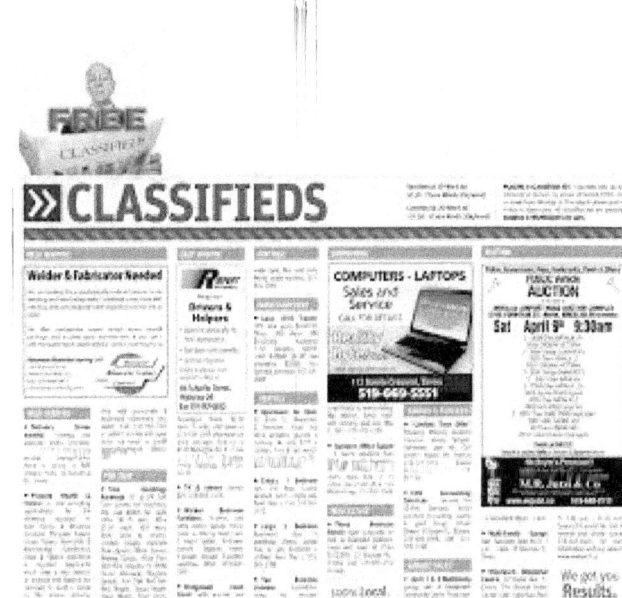

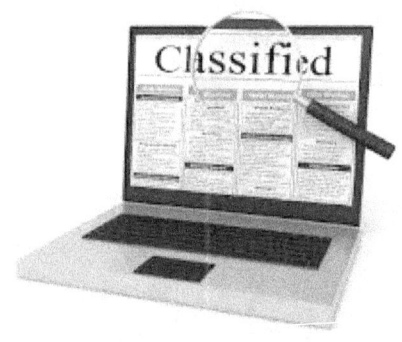

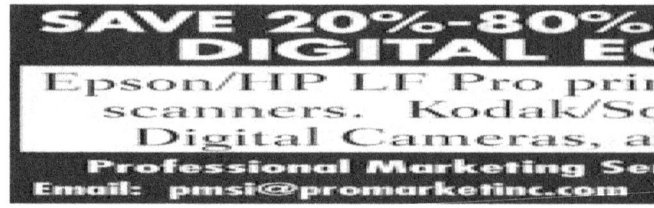
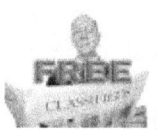

Home > for sale > furniture

## RESULTS FOR FURNITURE
## 1 - 30 OF 125

Sort by | Highest price first ▼

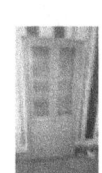

**Beechwood dresser cabinet in excellent condition**
Beechwood dresser cabinet in excellent condition. With 3 drawers and 3 glass shelves.
furniture5 days ago

$ 50

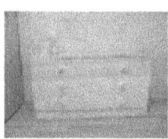

**white lowboy chest of drawers**
WHITE TIMBER LOWBOY GOOD CONDITION
furniture6 days ago

$ 160

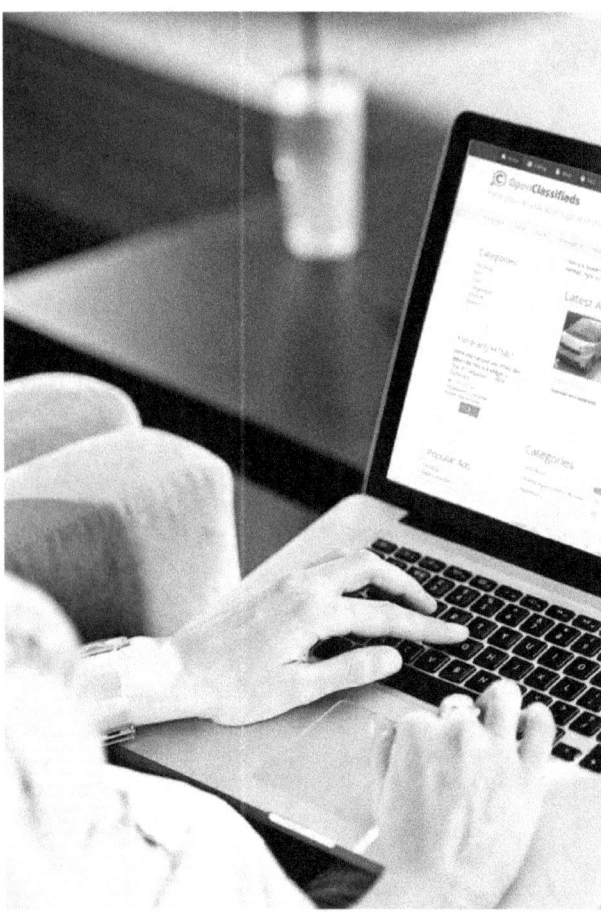

Classifieds are available everywhere, and in one place is your place where your next sell can be as easy as a one touch screen.

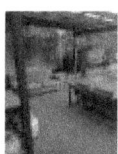

### Couch - free
Couch been outside under patio (no longer for inside) - some minor water staining; cleaning required; a small tear. Would be improved with a new cover/rug etc. Free to a good home.

furniture1 week ago

Free

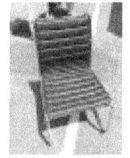

### Office chair
Good quality and good condition. 4 to choose from.

furniture1 week ago

$ 45

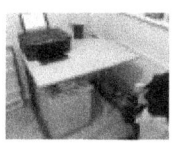

### Small computer desk
Ideal for a small corner to work from

furniture3 weeks ago

$ 0

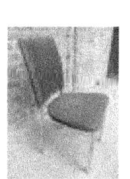

### 150 x CONFERENCE & BANQUETING CHAIRS
We have 150 x Conference & banqueting Chairs for sale. All in ok

Please contact

condition however because they are stored in a non heated warehouse the fabric has gone a little mouldy. Please be aware this is easily resolved as the...

furniture4 weeks ago

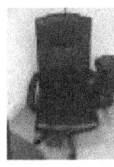

### Black office chair
Office chair in used but decent condition.

furniture4 weeks ago

### Beechwood dresser cabinet in excellent condition

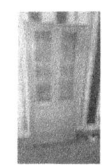

Beechwood dresser cabinet in excellent condition. With 3 drawers and 3 glass shelves.

$ 50

furniture5 days ago

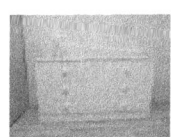

### white lowboy chest of drawers

WHITE

$ 160

TIMBER
LOWBOY
GOOD
CONDITION

**furniture**6 days ago

## Small computer desk

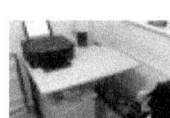

Ideal for a small corner to work from

$ 0

**furniture**3 weeks ago

## Couch - free

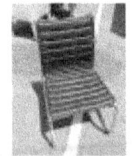

Couch been outside under patio (no longer for inside) - some minor water staining; cleaning required; a small tear. Would be improved with a new cover/rug etc. Free to a good home.

Free

**furniture**1 week ago

## 150 x CONFERENCE & BANQUETING CHAIRS

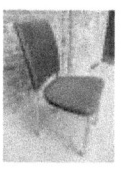

We have 150 x Conference & banqueting Chairs for sale. All in ok condition however because they are stored in a non heated warehouse the fabric has gone a little mouldy. Please be aware this is easily resolved as the...

Please contact

**furniture**4 weeks ago

## Office chair

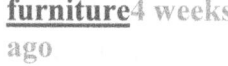

Good quality and good condition. 4 to choose from.

$ 45

**furniture**1 week ago

### Black office chair

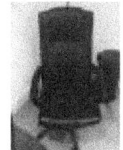

Office chair in used but decent condition. $ 15

**furniture**4 weeks ago

### Leksvik Desk for sale

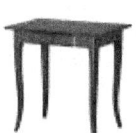

Hi there! I have moved house and need to get rid of some furniture quickly. I have a Leksvik desk that I want to sell. We can negotiate on price. I only used it for about 3 months so it's... $ 80

**furniture**9 weeks ago

### Kinnarps round office table

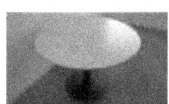

Kinnarps round office table. Very nice low profile metal base. The table top is a bit damages on the edge as it fell out of the van and $ 10 rolled down a hill before I caught up with it-...

**furniture**9 weeks ago

### Office organiser

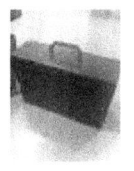

Needs to go asap. I have 2 very similar $ 10

**furniture**9 weeks ago

### Four quality thick solid wood tables

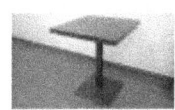

Four quality thick solid wood tables in great condition. Delivery can be arranged at competitive price. $ 20

**furniture**9 weeks ago

### Three quality stacking visitor chairs perfect condition

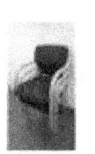

Three quality $ 10

stacking visitor chairs in perfect condition. Delivery available at competitive prices for multiple orders.

**furniture**9 weeks ago

### Large curved desk

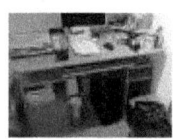

Great condition Easy removal as comes apart

$ 50

**furniture**14 weeks ago

### Techni-Mobili Workstation/Desk

Hi, I'm selling a used multi-purpose workstation, Italian design, high-quality, slick functionality, separate keyboard pull-out, high-rise corner shelf for

$ 50

stationary and plenty of room for monitor, desktop tower and/or hi-fi, needs to go to a good home as it's well...

**furniture**14 weeks ago

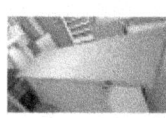

### Five desk partitions

I have five desk partition boards

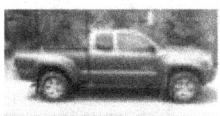

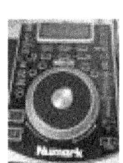
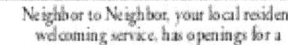
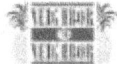
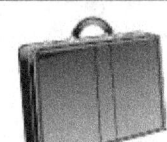
# RESULTS FOR MUSICAL INSTRUMENTS 1 - 30 OF 189

Sort by [ New listed ▼ ]

### Dj deck Numark NDX400
OVERVIEW FEATURES FAQPlay and scratch from MP3s, CDs and USB flash drives.NDX400 is an advanced, touch-activated scratch MP3/CD player that can also play from a USB flash drive. Numark's Anti-Shock™ buffered skip-protection technology keeps the music playing even when vibrations...
musical instruments 3 days ago

$ 190

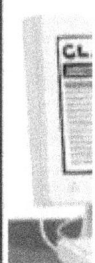

### Buffet alto saxophone
This is my lovely sax.Plays and sounds very nice . easy to play.and is all brass unlike some of the new one out there
musical instruments 3 weeks ago

$ 200

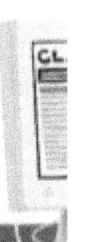

### AMYL Pianola, full size, for restoration
This Pianola is free to a good home. It needs some restoration, been in my garage for 4 years, so kept dry. New owner to collect please, It's heavy. Como of the keys are stiff, and some, if not all,...
musical instruments 4 weeks ago

Free

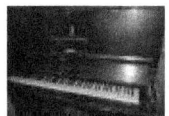

### Tokai GoldStar Sound electric guitar - S/type - Japan - 1980's - Red

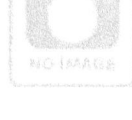

PRIVATE SELLER. COLLECTOR HAS FOR SALE. PRIVATE SELLER. Lovely red finished Tokai guitar from the 1980's. These guitars sold faster than the US product back in the 1980's. The quality of the Japanese craftsmanship was far superior than the...

musical instruments 4 weeks ago

$ 100

### YAMAHA PSR --170 ELECTRIC KEYBOARD

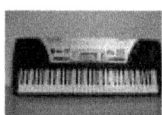

YAMAHA PSR--170 ELECTRIC KEYBOARD WITH SONG/STYLE/VOICE/PH ONES IN AND OUT/SUSTAIN/MMIDI IN AND OUT, IIT HAS A DJ SECTION WHEN DJ BUTTON IS ON IT PLAYS ALL SORT OF DJ SOUNDS, COMES WITH MAINS ADAPTER.

musical instruments 4 weeks ago

$ 50

### Pioneer CDJ 2000 mint

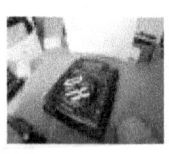

Pioneer CDJ 2000 Professional DJ Deck With Rekordbox software, Cables & Manuals. In mint condition, has never been gigged with only light practice at home.

musical instruments 7 weeks ago

$ 1000

### Gibson J-Series Replica Acoustic Guitar

Gibson J-Series Acoustic Guitar This guitar has been designed to offer the Gibson J-Series looks and most of the tone for a fraction of the cost. The guitar itself is more than 40 years old but has been...

musical instruments 8 weeks ago

$ 200

### Nord Electro 3 HP

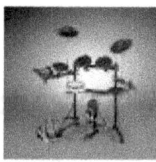

Nord Electro 3 HP 73 Keys 2 years old Not been used more than about ten times at home No marks or scratches Comes with 'The Nord Piano Library V5' CD And Also Yamaha Sustainer...

musical instruments 9 weeks ago

$ 1200

### Casio Midi Guitar

watch you the youtube video! just plug and play! PERFECT FOR GUITARISTS COMPOSING SOUNDTRACKS. A truely rare and special guitar with midi controller. An incredible composing, recording and performance tool. You won't see another one of these turn...

musical instruments 9 weeks ago

$ 600

### Roland TD-6KV vdrum kit with pedal.

Mesh Snare and Dual-Trigger Cymbals Please note - the kit on offer is the same as in the home pictures and the last one (slight differences). The frame is the updated MDS-

$ 500

6C with curved tubes and in gunmetal...

musical instruments 9 weeks ago

### BOSS CH-1 Guitar Pedal - All Analogue Pink Label Edition

Boxed guitar chorus effects pedal.BOSS CH-1 Super Chorus - Rare 90's Analogue Pink Label Version - Good condition just a couple of light knocks (see the pic), works flawlessly.

$ 50

musical instruments 10 weeks ago

### Yamaha tyros 2 with speakers and 40 gb hard drive

yamaha tyros 2 instrumet in exelent condition working perfect, really beautifull voices low price!!!!

$ 700

musical instruments 13 weeks ago

### FULL DJ SETUP FOR SALE

Full DJ setup all in perfect working condition a little bit of damage to 1 speaker but still works perfectly I have used it for 2years and just haven't got the time to do party's or karaoke

$ 600

musical instruments 14 weeks ago

### Peavey Bandit 112 guitar amp

Very loud 100w Guitar Amp supplied with a foot switch to select between channels from crisp clean to a wicked distortion this amp delivers a great sound

Please contact

for any budding guitarist (make a nice Christmas present ) at I believe...

musical instruments 14 weeks ago

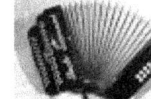

### Paolo Soprani B/C button accordion Black 4 voice

Paolo Soprani professional instrument! Needs nothing. 4 voice,2 treble registers,8 bass! The tuning is perfect. Rare to find a Paolo Soprani in black! Any questions feel to call!

$ 1300

musical instruments 15 weeks ago

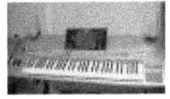

### Stagg mandolin

Stagg mandolin. As good as new. Only played a few times.

$ 40

musical instruments 15 weeks ago

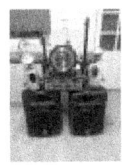

### yamaha tyros 1

hi. i have yamaha tyros 1 for sale is in good condition played only at home but i do not have speakers .

$ 500

musical instruments 16 weeks ago

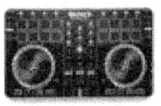

### Numark MixTrack Pro II 2 Channel DJ Controller 3 months old

Here i have for sale the numark mixtrack pro 2 its in really good condition and comes with box etc. This is the worlds number 1 dj controller and would be a must for any budding or intermediate dj or...

$ 120

musical instruments 17 weeks ago

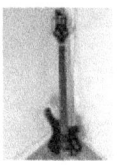

### 2 guitars cheap cheap
2 guitars Selling because im cleaning my storage and need space
musical instruments18 weeks ago

$ 150

### Soprano Saxophone (As New)

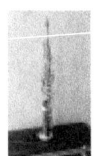

Soprano Saxophone by "Gear For Music". 2 necks, new unused reeds, new, unused "chilli pepper" neck strap, rigid flight case, everything required. Purchased with a view to learning, but never got round to it. Has been out it's case maybe...
musical instruments18 weeks ago

Please contact

### PRS Custom 22 2013

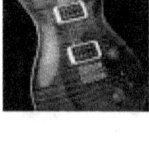

Stunning PRS Custom 22 2013 Model in Grey/Black. Recently purchased but has mainly remained in the case due to me not having much time to play. Immaculate condition, a dream to play and sounds fantastic! Pickups are Vintage Bass and...
musical instruments19 weeks ago

$ 0

### 2 guitar.s for sale swap or trade
for sale swap trade or part ex 2 ov my guitars for a gibson country style acoustic guitar or an epiphone j300 country jumbo acoustic my guild gad 40p performer in solid mahogany body back side,s & solid top amazeing...
musical instruments20 weeks

$ 1000

ago

### FENDER CLASSIC PLAYER BAJA TELECASTER HONEY BLONDE

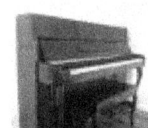

Beautiful guitar, sorry to see it go, but can't justify having so many guitars. his sounds and is built like an American Telecaster IMHO. Has S Switch for more tonal options. Plays fast and sounds gorgeous. One year old, selling...
musical instruments35 weeks ago

$ 400

### KARL MULLER UPRIGHT PIANO
Karl Muller upright piano for sale. Beautiful condition. Mahogany with matching piano stool
musical instruments40 weeks ago

$ 1500

### Acoustic Guitar & Sealed Guitar Starter Pack for Sale
Perfect present for beginners. Full size. Black. Beautiful shape. Will throw in: - brand new black guitar carry bag and strap, guitar plectrum & extra steel strings. - sealed `The Essential Series Guitar Starter Pack`: ...
musical instruments40 weeks ago

$ 150

### Line 6 POD HD 500 - Pristine Condition - All Original Bits Included
Selling my POD HD 500 multieffect floor unit. Bought a year and a half ago, hardly ever used (only in my flat) so the condition

$ 290

is absolutely amazing. It is all in its original packaging, complete with power adapter,...

musical instruments40 weeks ago

### Roland V-Studio 20 for sale

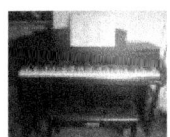

Cakewalk by Roland V-STUDIO 20 audio interface/control surface for sale. Unit is only 6 months old, boxed and in mint condition. All software is included, and is compatible with most modern DAWs. Unit rarely used, hence the reason for...

musical instruments41 weeks ago

Please contact

### FENDER STRATOCASTER MIM

Bought new in 1997. Honey sunburst with maple fingerboard. White pearl scratchplate and upgraded pick-ups. Almost mint. Great looks and sound. Professionally set up with 10-52 Elixir strings. Includes hard case.

$ 400

musical instruments41 weeks ago

### Amazing digital piano

I am selling a fantastic digital piano. It's barely been used and it is in a perfect condition. It has 88 weighted touch responsive keys. Feels same as a not digital piano but you can play with headphones, external speakers...

$ 400

musical instruments44 weeks ago

### Squier Classic Vibe Stratocaster

Squier Classic Vibe Stratocaster for sale. It's in perfect condition and recently restrung with 10's. An amazing sounding guitar that could easily compete with Mexican made Fender Strats!

$ 175

musical instruments44 weeks ago

Home > for sale > health, beauty, special needs

# Results for health, beauty, special needs 1 - 9 of 9

Sort by
| New listed ▼ |
|---|

### MAC make up, brand new never been used or even touched

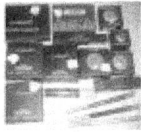

They are brand new and unwanted gift to me, and I didnot use this brand, so I want to buy my brand that I usually use,,And if u near, we

Please contact

### Hearing aid batteries #312

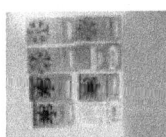

I have 13 packs totaling 78 #312 batteries for $13. Each pack has 6 batteries. Expiration date is 6-14 or 5-15.

$ 1

health, beauty, special needs0 sec

# My Connections Magazine

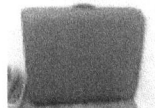

### Massage table
Earth lite Avalon massage table, teal, 32 lbs., mint condition, carrying case included, head rest, max wt 700. Lbs, high quality 3" multi layer foam, 30" x 70.

$ 200

health, beauty, special needs0 sec

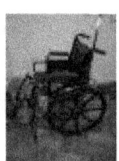

### Wheelchair, Great Condition
I am selling this wheelchair since we have no use for it anymore, its honestly just taking up space. I know nothing of wheelchairs but feel free to ask me any questions you may have. Price is negotiable*

$ 300

health, beauty, special needs0 sec

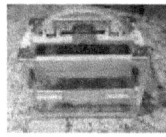

### Sephora Make Up Case
Sephora Make Up Case 2. Email me if interested.

$

health, beauty, special needs0 sec

# WORLD'S 3 BEST BEACHES TO VISIT IN 2015!

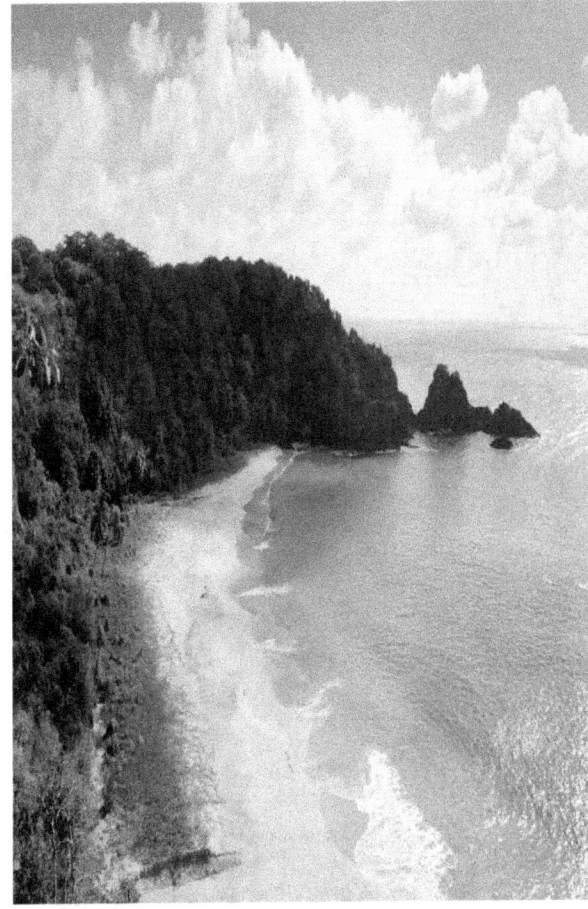

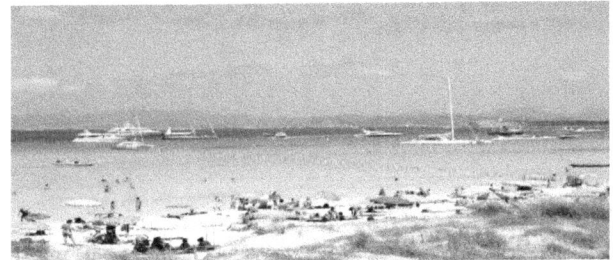

**1. Baia do Sancho, Fernando de Noroha, Brazil**

Drumroll please... The very best beach in the world lives in Brazil and goes by the name of Baia do Sancho.

### 2. Grace Bay, Providenciales, Turks and Caicos

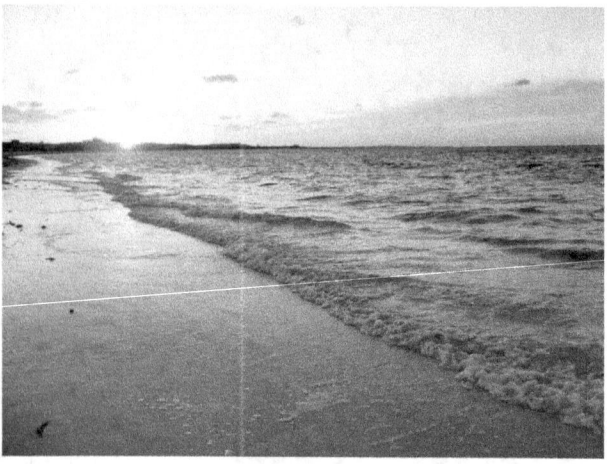

This is basically one of the most perfect Caribbean beaches you will ever have the pleasure of sunbathing on. Temperatures are delightful all year round so feel free to visit any time you like.

### 3. Rabbit Beach, Lampedusa, Italy

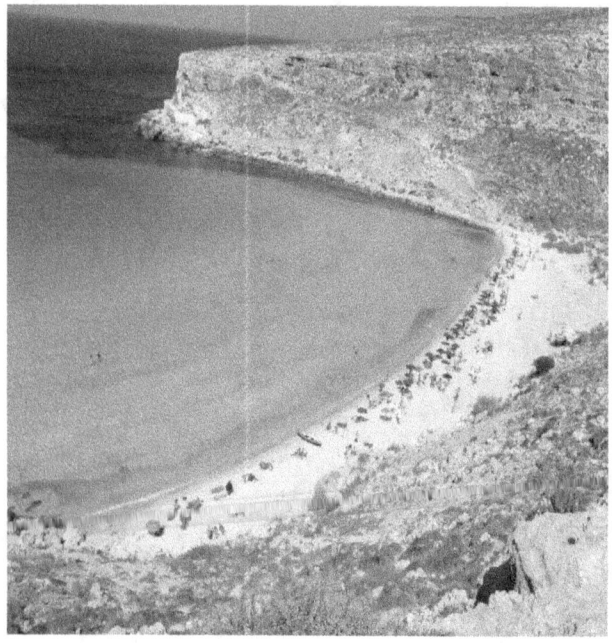

Closer to Tunisia than to Italy's mainland, Rabbit Beach is a little slice of Meditteranean

# Best looking six pack Abs Real Stuff..Real

#3

#3

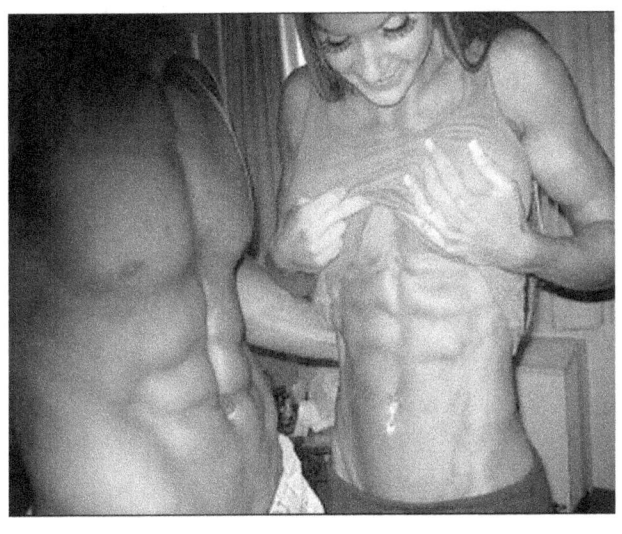

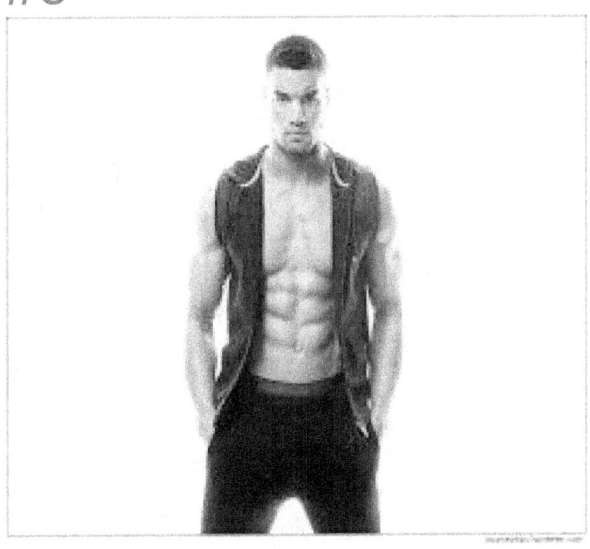

#2

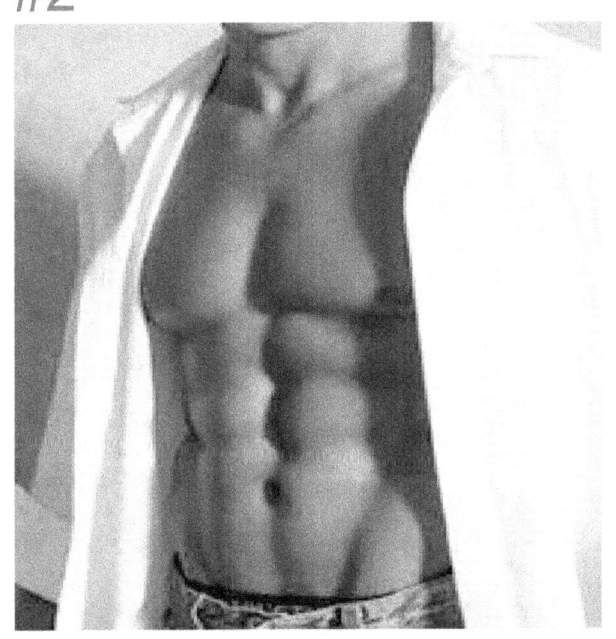

Dude..in the kitchen

Where to begin. Lean cuisine. Eat lean…

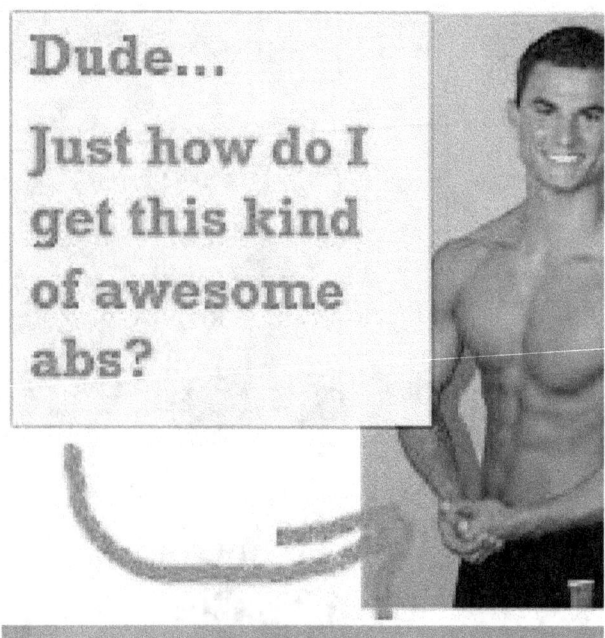

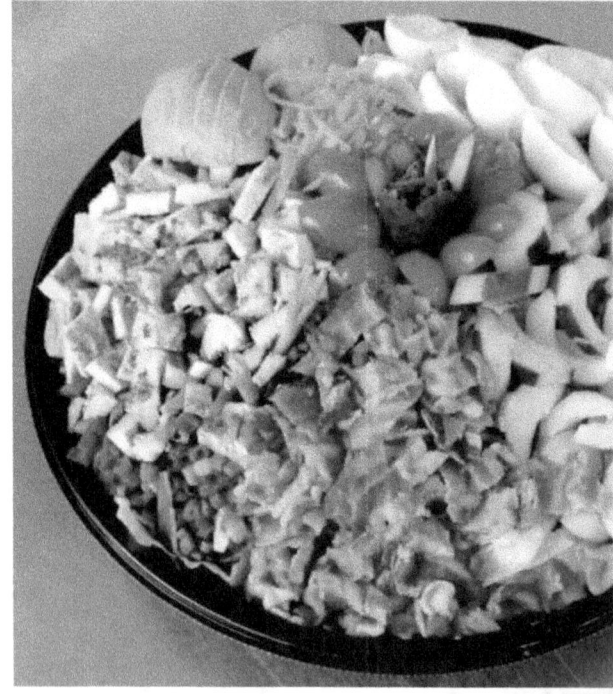

# SELECT A CATEGORY So MUCH AVAILABLE FREE

## services
- music lessons
- moving, storage
- entertainment
- fitness, personal trainer
- financial, legal
- babysitter, nanny
- wedding
- cleaners, cleaning
- computer
- painters, painting
- photography, video
- health, beauty
- tutors, languages
- other

## housing
- apartment for rent
- house for rent
- room rental, roommates
- commercial
- housing for sale
- vacation rentals
- short term rentals
- real estate services
- other

## for sale
- computers
- computer accessories
- home appliances
- cameras, camcorders
- baby items
- jewellery, watches
- cds, dvds, vhs
- musical instruments
- video games, consoles, toys
- books
- hobbies, crafts
- furniture
- tools, equipment
- health, beauty, special needs
- sports, bikes
- phones, PDAs
- MP3 players, ipods
- clothing, accessories
- Tv, accessories
- other

## cars & vehicles
- cars
- motorcycles

- parts, accessories
- automotive services
- SUVs, trucks, vans

jobs
- office mgr, receptionist
- bar, food, hospitality
- non profit sector
- driver-security
- hair stylist, salon
- accounting-mgmt
- construction, trades
- child care
- cleaning, housekeeper
- programmers, computer
- customer service
- part time, students
- general labour
- tv, media, fashion
- sales, retail sales
- graphic, web design
- other

personals
- long lost relationships
- just friends
- casual encounters
- women seeking men
- women seeking women
- men seeking women
- men seeking men
- missed connections

Business Directory

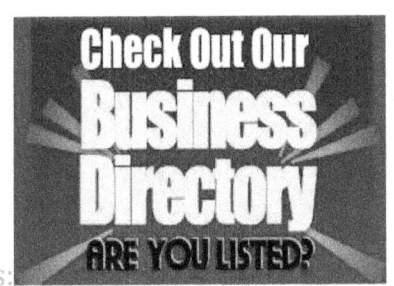

Categories:

Connections Magazine at myconnectionsmagazine.com and at weconnect2.com

Listing your business in the Business Directory promote and engage your business daily activities in a broad market place.

One step into getting to know other businesses who might need your services, and your business need could be in that one listing next to your business name.

Our Services are magic. Yes there is magic in advertising and marketing your business while you sit back and relax and enjoy a busy day with customers or visitors you have not targeted.

We mean Connections because we have been connecting Buyers and Sellers for over 10 years. Sure we are asking something in return and everything is not free. We are like your business looking to maximize our customers base.

We connect buyers and sellers with every possible opportunity available,

If you have a suggestions please forward to our email

Weconnect2@live.com

## Arts and crafts

Hampshire Traders

An online store selling oil paintings and other works of art.

http://www.hampshiretraders.com

Automobile

Interstateautoclub

club members have it all, towing, insurance, auto show, and advertising.
http:www.interstateautoclub.co


Business

weconnect2media

public relation, group of companies producing, publishing, and education outreach.
http//:www.weconnect2.com


Arizona Business Professionals

Search a directory of Arizona business professionals including Lawyers, Accountants, Architects, Realtors, and more.
http://www.azbizpros.com


Blue Boomerang - Business Directory

Search the Blueboomerang directory guide for a wide range of business listings covering a variety of areas.
http://www.blueboomerang.comt


Business Directory

Local Search 24 is a business directory for the Norfolk region. The directory lists many businesses from many different industries.
http://www.localsearch24.co.uk

eMetro411 Houston Texas

An information portal and business directory for residents and small business owners in Houston Texas.

http://www.emetro411.com

Fuzing.com

An international business to business (b2b) trade portal that helps buyers and suppliers of goods and services to overcome the major hurdle of locating suitable trading partners.

http://www.fuzing.com

Houston Business Directory

A web directory for Houston businesses who need to advertise their website on the internet and web.

http://www.houston-area.com

Investing In China

Submit and read new investment and business opportunities in China, consult a directory of Chinese manufacturers and investment companies.

http://www.investinginchina.co.uk

Careers

policewithoutborders
police community news and feud, public relation, and multimedia advertising.
http//:www.policewithoutborders.com
Computer

Education
National Universe Students Journal
college and universities studens participation in the community.
http//:www.nusjournal
Entertainment

**World Mentoring Academy**
FREE Interactive Learning OpenCourseware
from MIT, UC Berkeley, Harvard, Yale, Stanford, U Houston, USC, UCLA, Khan ...
http//:www.worldmentoringacademy.com

Health and Fitness

Fitness First Gyms, Download Free Pass

Get a free Fitness First gym pass and check out gym membership offers at the local gym.

http://www.fitnessfirst.co.uk/

Garmin Edge 500

Athleti offers a range of endurance sports equipment including some of the latest Garmin products.

http://www.athleti.ca

## Health and Fitness

Tennis, gyms, swimming, wet spas and more at the UK based David Lloyd Leisure Group health and fitness club.

http://www.davidlloyd.co.uk/

## Klick Fitness

fitness club, Klick Fitness have several gyms throughout the UK with cardiovascular and strength training machines available.

http://www.klickfitness.com

## Personal Trainer Richmond Hill

Toronto Fitness Online offers personal training sessions around the Greater Toronto area.

http://www.torontofitnessonline.com/

## Health and fitness sports magazine

online magazine featuring articles, advertising, events, and resources for sports and recreation,**fitness** and exercise, **health** and wellness.

www.healthfitnessmag.com

Home and Garden

## visions in furniture

experience, personable, value

all your furniture needs.
http//:www.visionsinfurnitureinc.com

Law Offices

You can trust the experience of our office when deciding to file for bankruptcy. Whether it is a Chapter 7 bankruptcy to eliminate credit card debt, or a Chapter 13 bankruptcy to help save your home from foreclosure and eliminate a second mortgage - See more at::
http://aibrahimlaw.com/

Lifestyle and Romance

Money and Finance

Publishing

Anaheim Publishing

custom publishing and media, books online, articles and short stories, press releasses, advertising online, special design of marketing and advertising campaign materials on line.

http//:www.anaheimpublishing.co
Reference

**Custom publishing**

custom media, & Custom magazines for high impact branding & relationship marketing. Exclusive distribution channels for B2B marketing.
http//:www.custompublishingne.com

Society

Sports

Sport Business Digestt
sport news online. uptodate ranking of sport figures.
*hhtp//::wwww.sportsbusinessdigest.com*

Toys Games

Travel
http//:www.hotwire.com/
Tripadvisor_Reviews of

hotels, flights and vacation Rentals
unbiased hotel reviews, photos and travel advice for hotels and vacations.

www.hotwire.com/

Please submit your business information on this business directory page. We are improving the way we connect you to the network. Thank you for participating.

Connections Magazine at myconnectionsmagazine.com is a Publication of : weconnect2.com . We connect buyers+sellers, and visa versa.

From News U.S. Journal at nusjournal.com Adselect is the support services and advertising category.

Adselect is a stream of advertising from choices of good services in the community.

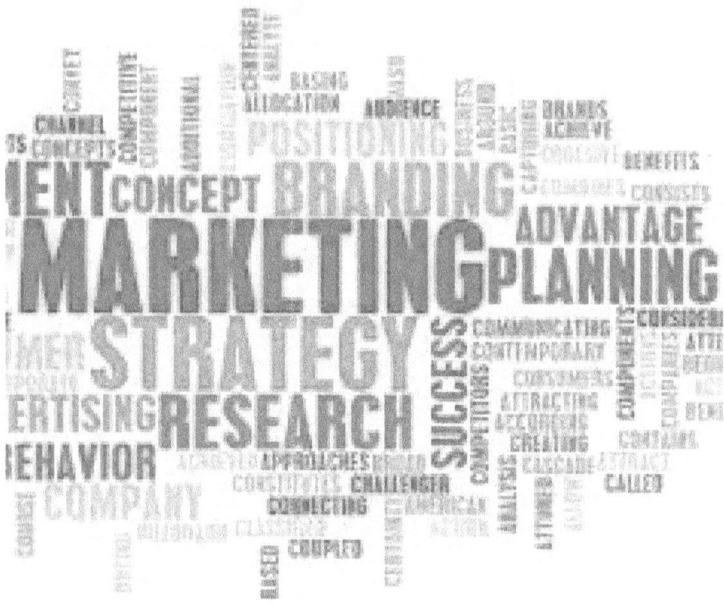

## ADSELECT- FAB PLACES AND GOODIES AROUND US…..

News U.S. Journal Support Services and Advertising.at nusjournal.com:

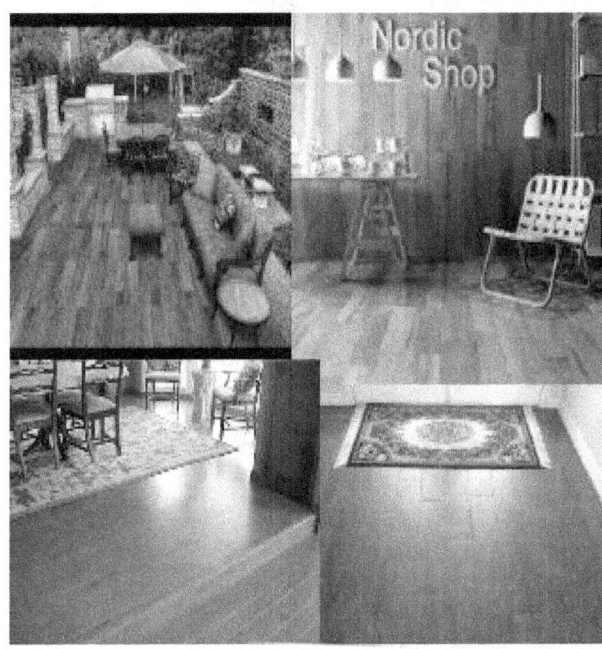

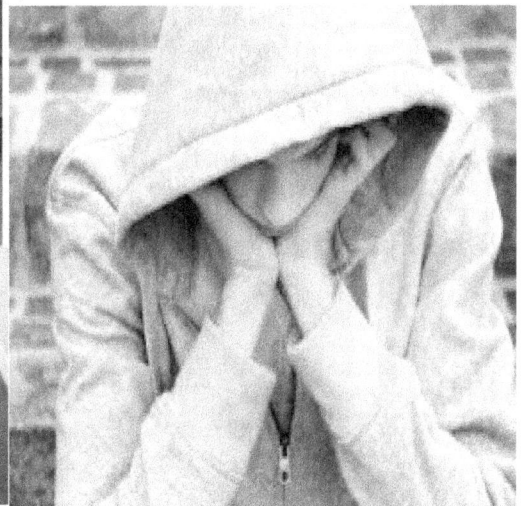

STAND UP FOR KIDS {888) 365-4543 COMMITMENT TO AMERICA AT-RISK YOUTH...IF YOU OR SOMEONE YOU KNOW IS BEING ABUSED, PLEASE CALL 1-800 4 ACHILD 1-800 422-4453

IF YOU HAVE RUN AWAY, OR THINKING ABOUT RUNNING AWAY, PLEASE CALL: 1-800 RUN AWAY 1-800 786-2929

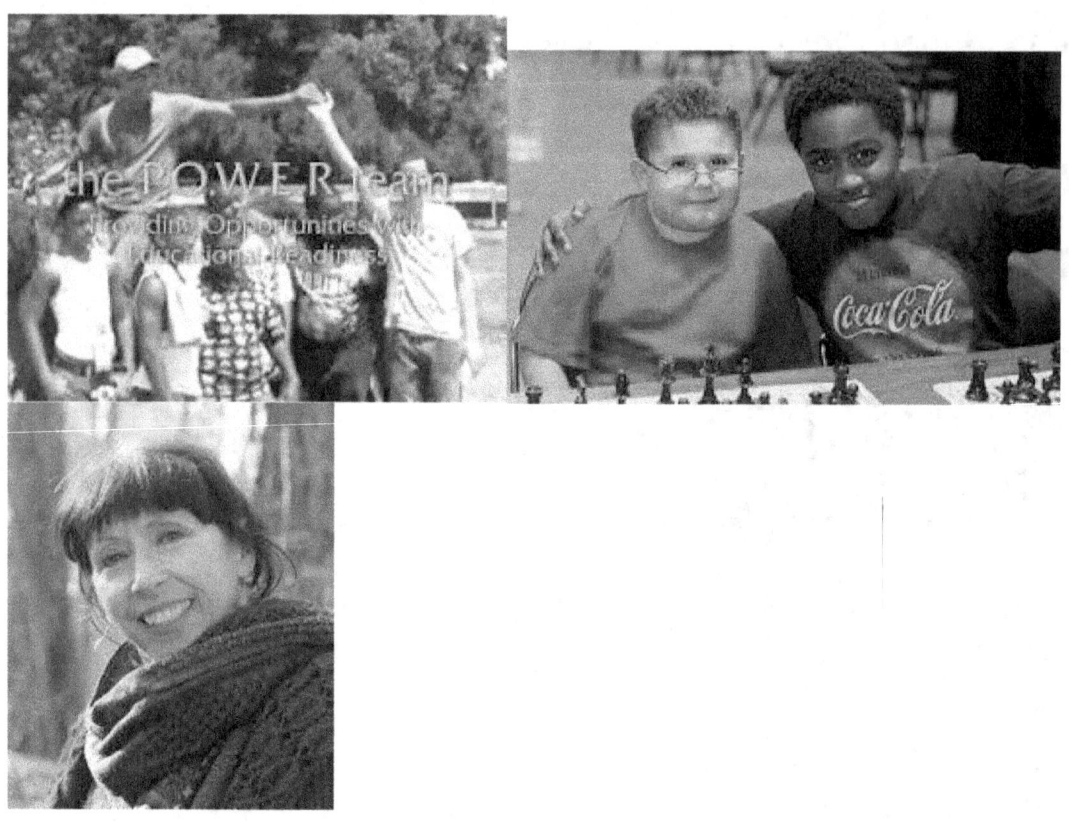

the P.O.W.E.R. team

YOUTH AT RISK – INTER-AMERICAN DEVELOPMENT BANK

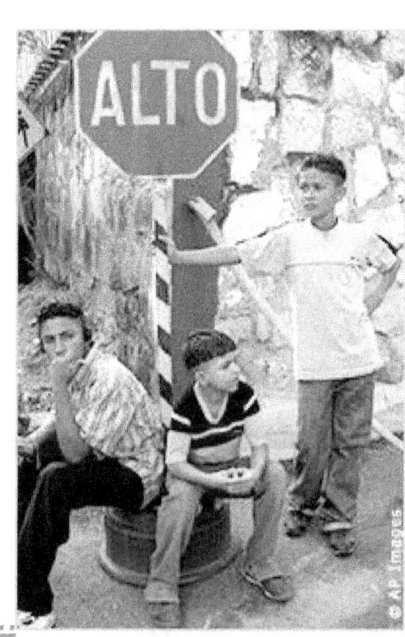

WARNING SIGNS OF YOUTH VIOLENCE – AMERICAN PSYCHOLOGICAL …

IT IS ABOUT QUALITY AND VALUE.  FRESH CHOICE HAVE IT

## *PITA HOT – A MIDDLE EASTERN GEM!*

Pita Hot is a Middle Eastern / Mediterranean restaurant that specializes in affordable meals that you can eat quickly. This place is one of those hidden gems that you would not expect to find in Fullerton, CA! You wont be disappointed in whatever you order (make sure to try the humus!) and your wallet wont be disappointed either. Though the service is a little slow, its more than worth it when the food finally arrives steaming hot and freshly made from the kitchen. You can tell the cooks and owners care about their food quality and ingredients they use in their dishes. Its a very casual place, so no need to feel bad going in there with your PJ's during finals! One of the best parts of this place is the amount of food you get. Each plate they serve is over flowing with food and the quality is superb. If your crunched for time and cant spend the time eating in the restaurant, they also do phone orders and take it, so you can take it back to your dorm, house, school, etc... All in all, a great place to go if your hungry for some Middle Eastern food and don't want to break the bank.

*1343 E Chapman Ave*
*Fullerton, CA 92831*

(714) 449-0100

http://www.pita-hot.com/

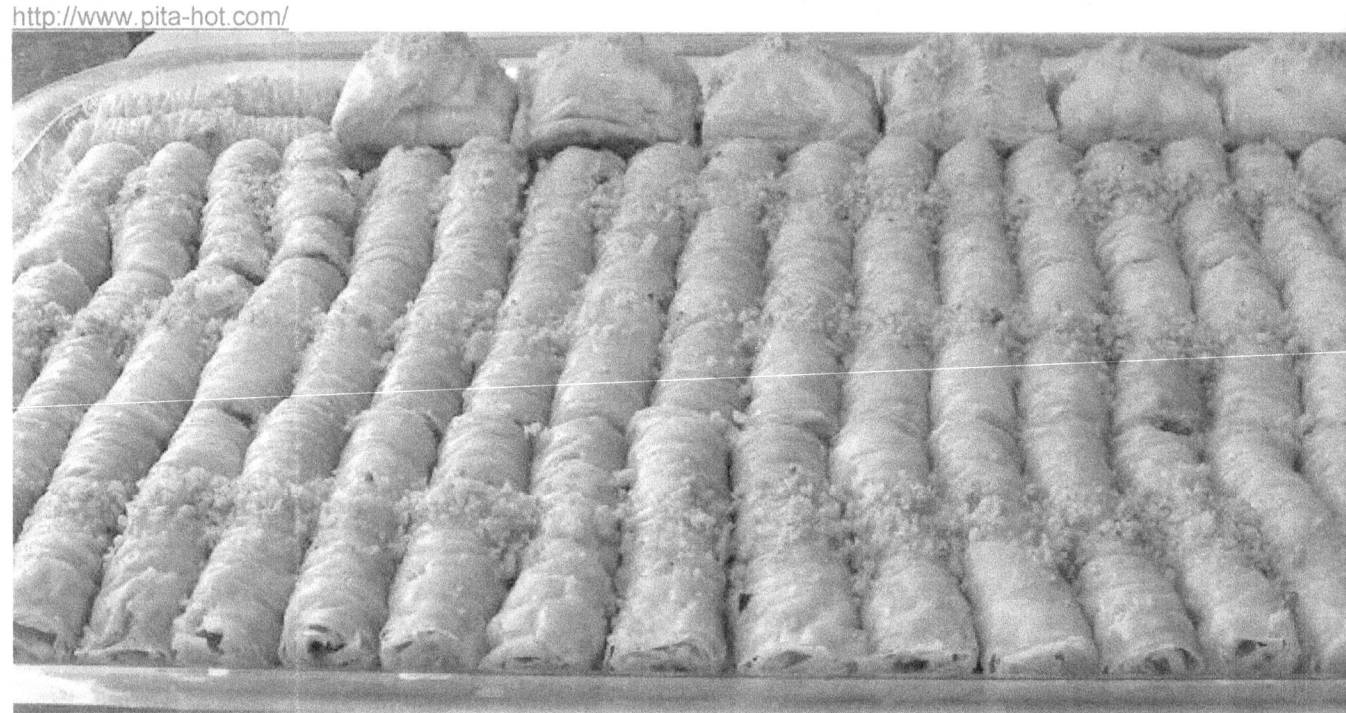

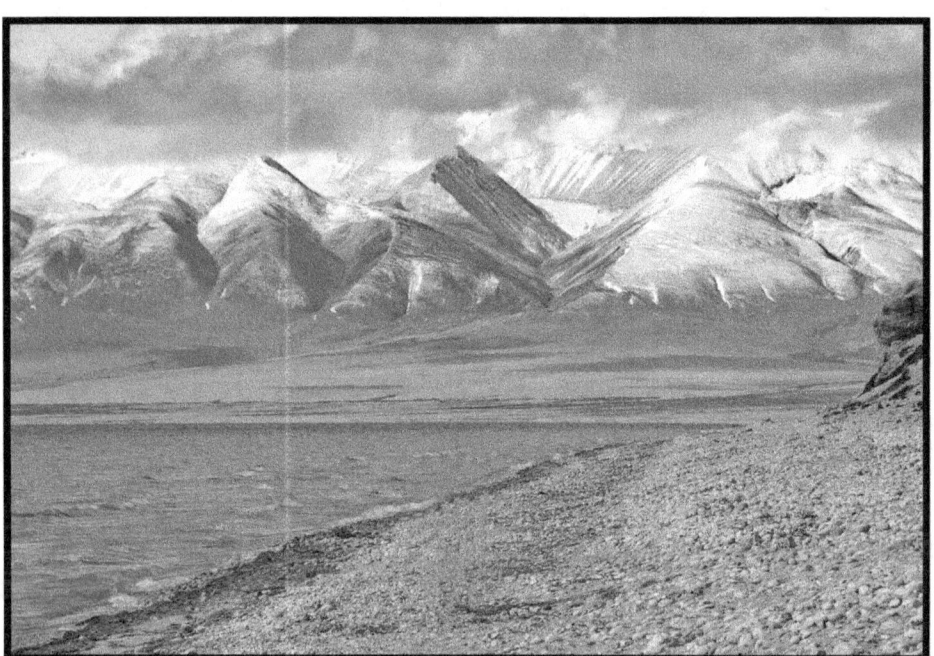

*MIKA AT panoramio.com ARTPHOTOGRAPHY......A TALENT CALLED ART.......*

# \* SUNSET CLIFFS ARTPHOTO......

World • United States • California

San Diego

Chat with mika online or call (858) 967-0891 art design, buy digital, consultant, adviser, ask for an appointment with MIKA TO GO OVER YOUR ART PROJECT....REASONABLE, FAIR, VALUE

YOU TOO LIKE A GREAT PHOTO OF YOUR HOUSE, LOVE ONE, OR YOUR SERVICE PET. EMAIL CMILTON111@GMAIL.COM

*INDULGE YOURSELF WITH OUR SOUTH OF THE BORDERS BEST. IF YOU ARE VISITING THE ANAHEIM AND GARDEN GROVE RESORTS, WE ARE AS CLOSE TO THE MEXICAN CULTURE AS ONE CAN GET. COME ON IN, OR ORDER BY PHONE OR ONLINE, AND ENJOY OUR FRESH MEXICAN FOOD.*

*BUENA COMIDA, MI CASA.......*

MI CASA MEXICANA RESTAURANT

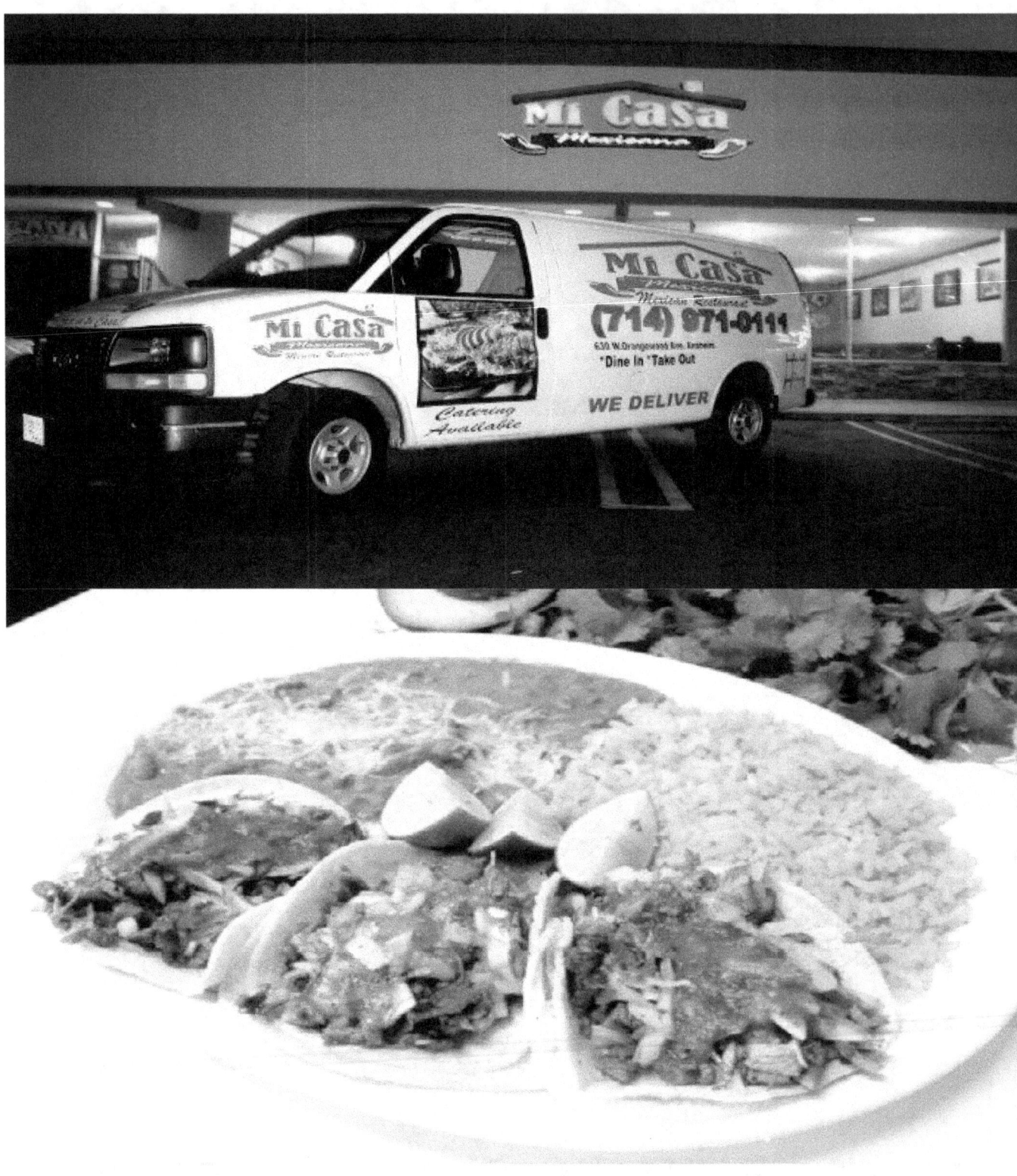

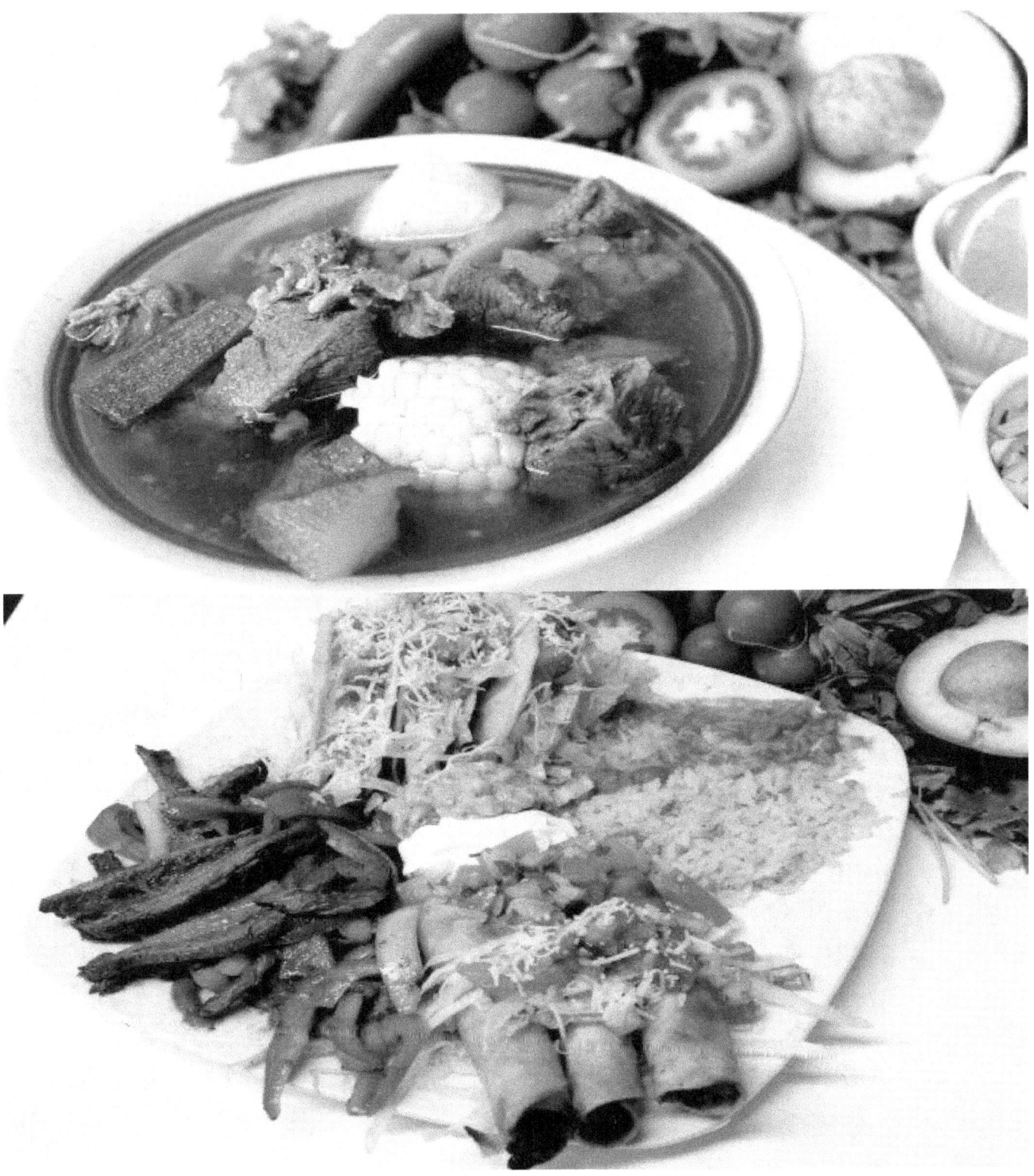

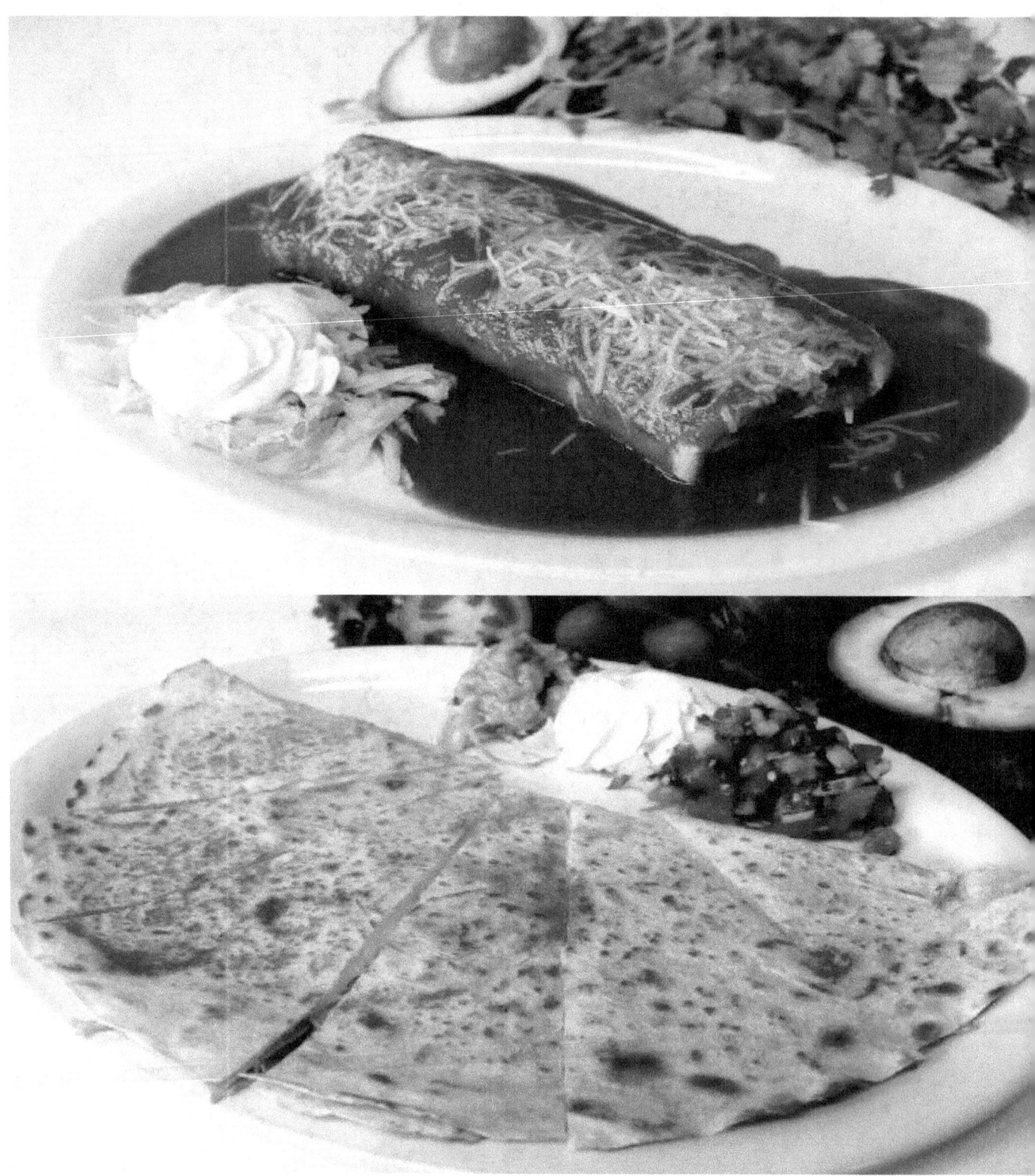

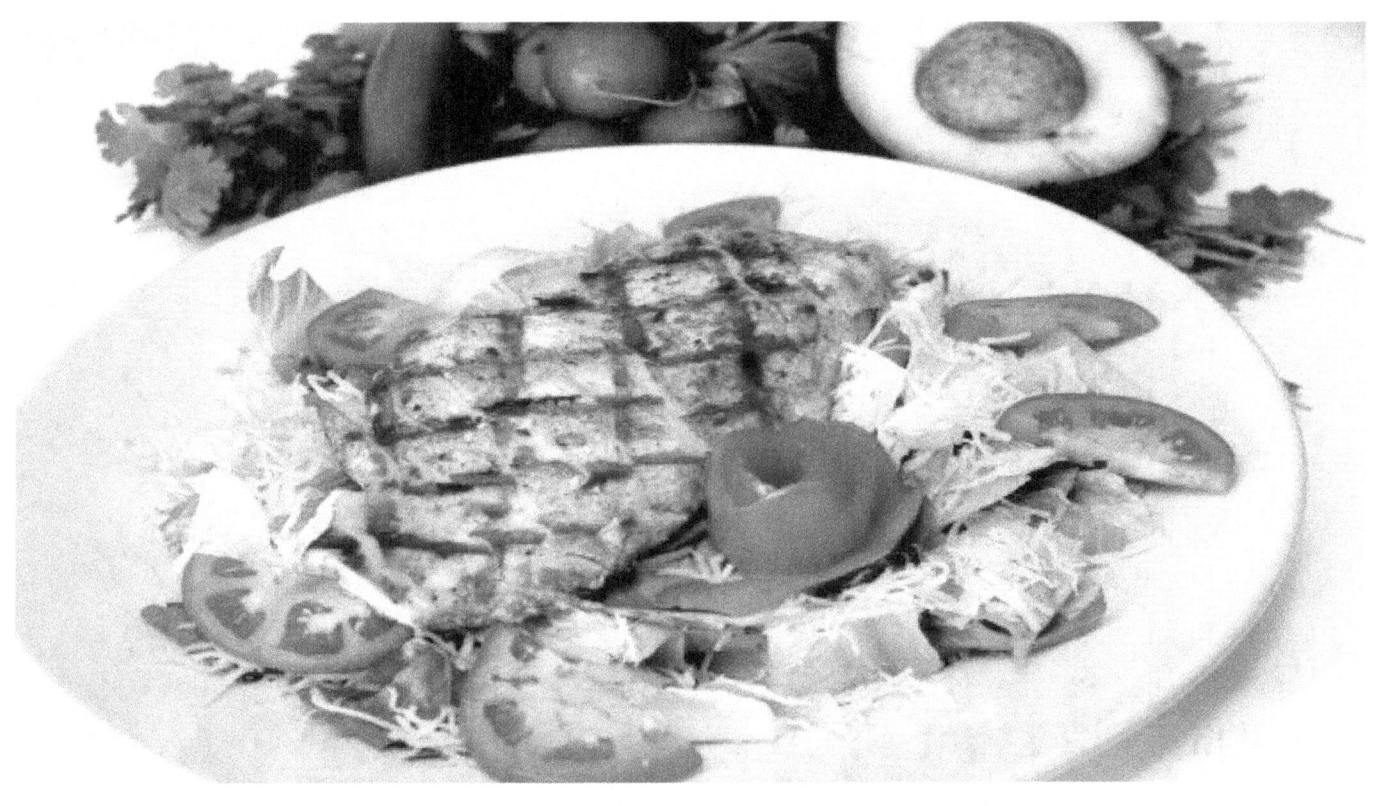

Address: 630 W. Orangewood Ave. Anaheim, CA 92802 | Phone: 714-971-0111 | Everyday: 11-10pm. Fri/Sat: 11-11pm.

FacebookYelp

COMING SOON """"MY CONNECTIONS MAGAZINE""""" SUMMER 14.........FOR ALL YOUR SPONSORED ADVERTISEMENTS, ANNOUNCEMENTS, AND PUBLIC NOTICE. CONTACT THE PUBLISHER..eddieadel@weconnect2.com 716 201-0012

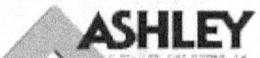

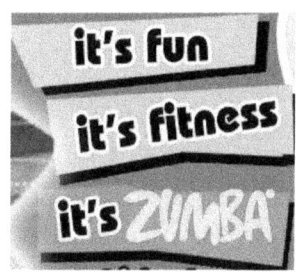

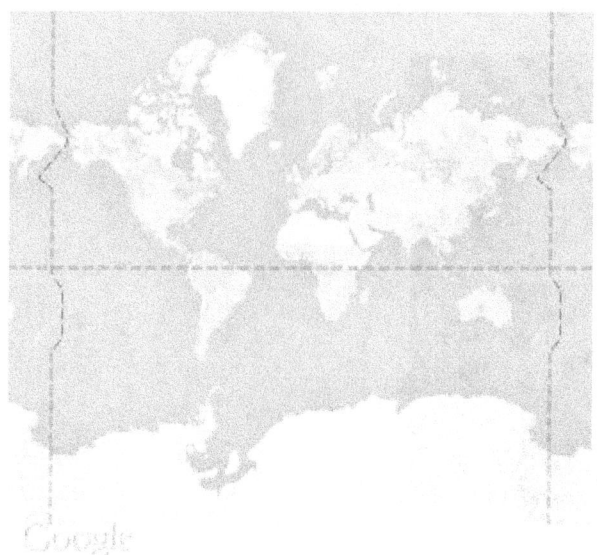

markers=icon%3Ahttp%3A%2F%2Fchart.googleapis.com%2Fchart%3Fchld%3D1%257C82b548%257Cffffff%26
chst%3Dd_map_pin_letter%7C33.7884407%2C-117.9237061" alt="" width="214" height="238" />

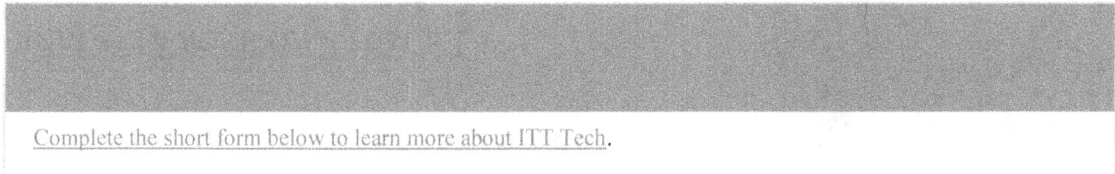

Complete the short form below to learn more about ITT Tech.

## FARMERS INSURANCE ANAHEIM, BILL DALATI

791 S Brookhurst St # 1

92804 Anaheim

CA

Phone:

(714) 956-2222

Fax:

(714) 956-2434

Website:

www.farmersagent.com/bdalati

We Give Personalized Quotes That Fit Your Budget; In Just 24 Hours!www.selectquote.com

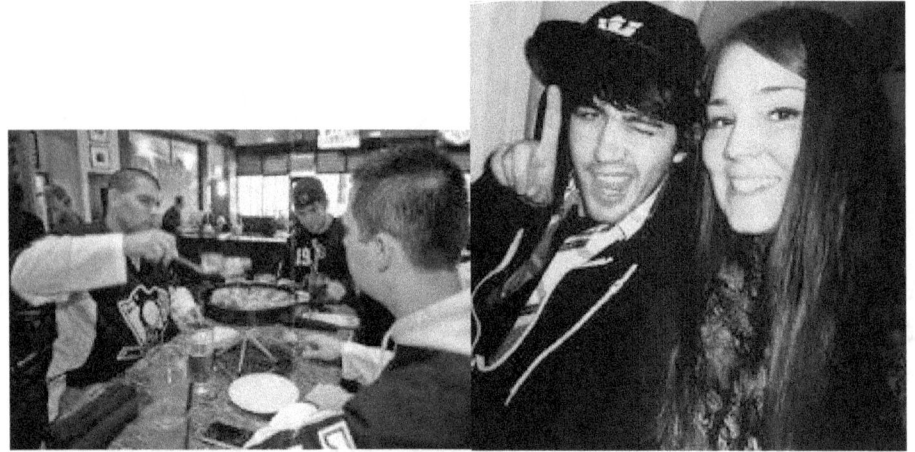

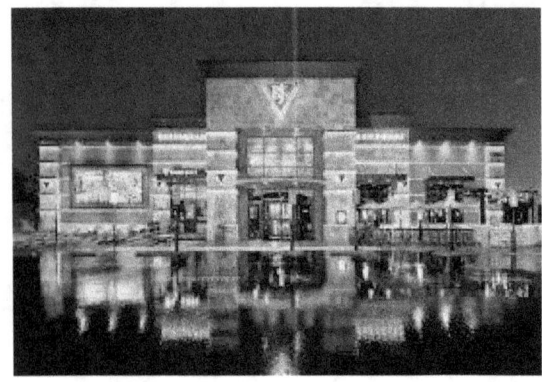

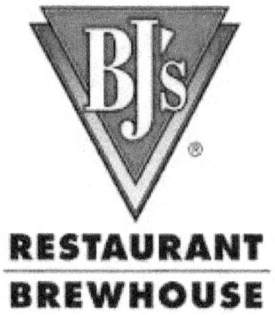

# HI-CREST LIQUOR & JUNIOR MARKET

- 12055 Chapman Ave
- Get Directions

- Phone number(714) 971-5463

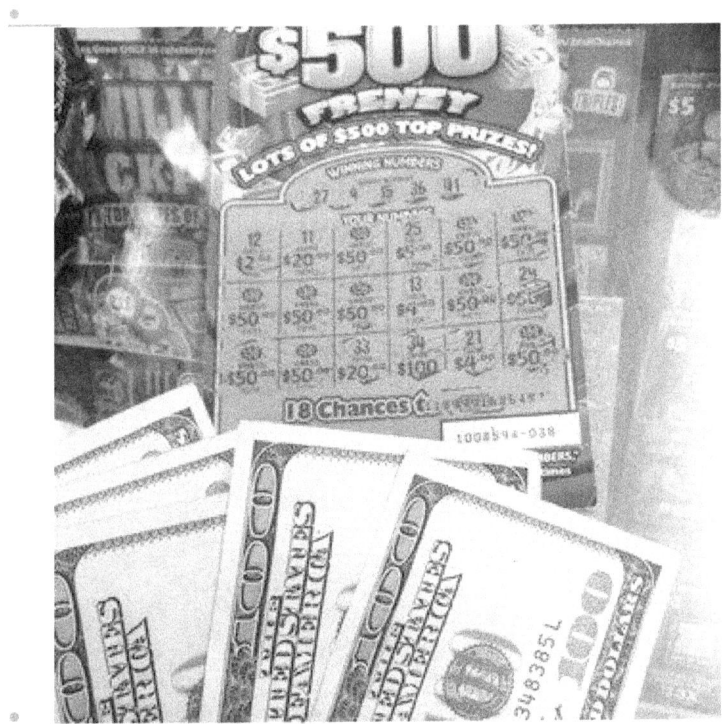

**Winners are sold here!**

Winners are sold here!

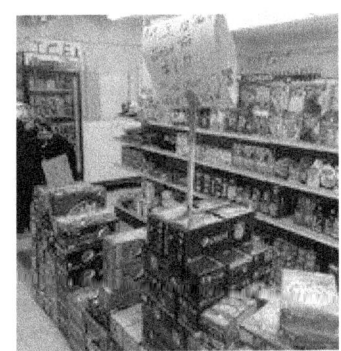

**ANY 12 pack 3 for 9**

ANY 12 pack 3 for 9

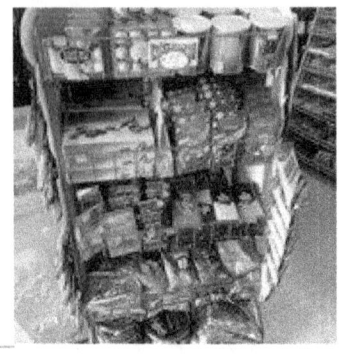

Great holiday deals! Only at hi crest!

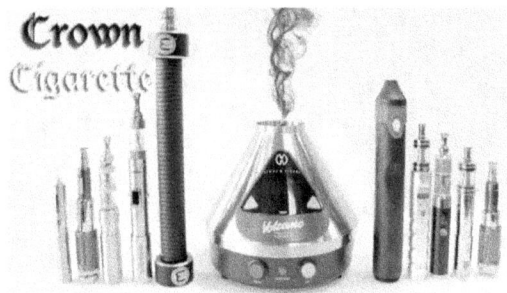

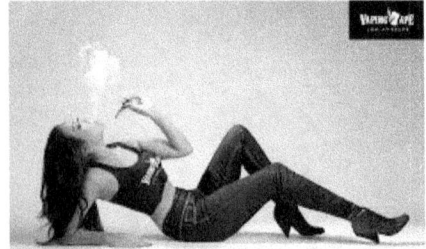

LITTLE SAIGON

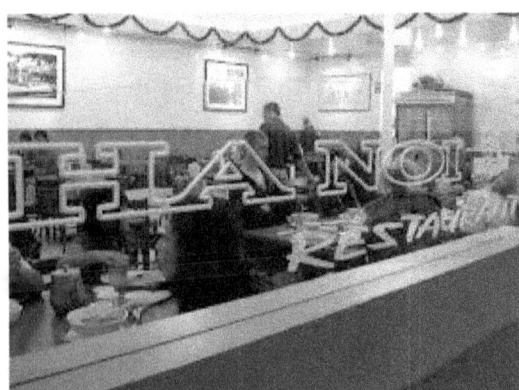

gastronomyblog.com Search by image

December 23, 2007. Cuisine: Vietnamese. 9082 Bolsa Avenue Westminster, CA 92683. Phone: 714-901-8108.
Website: http://www.hanoirest.com/index.html

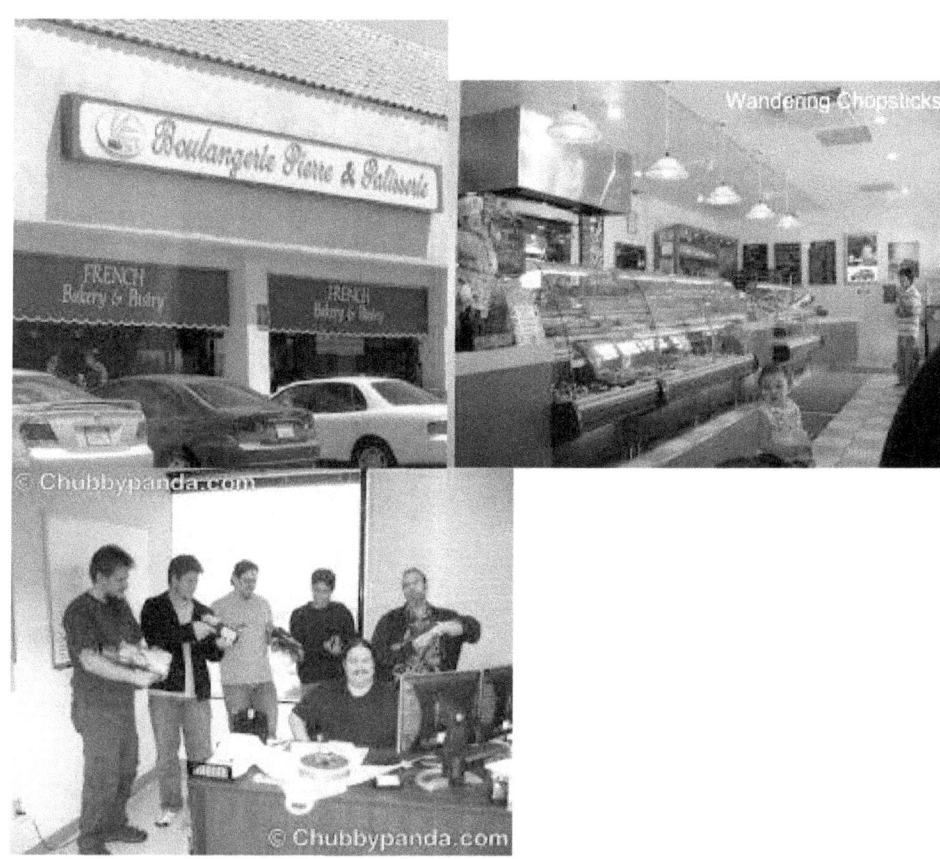

## BOULANGERIE PIERRE & PATISSERIE – GARDEN GROVE, CA

14352 Brookhurst St, Garden Grove, CA 92843. Directions ....

++++++++++++++++++++++++++++++++++++++++++++++++++++++++++++++++++++++++++++++++++++++++

Advertising examples of internet and e bus

We Deliver at Thai Little Home

We Deliver!

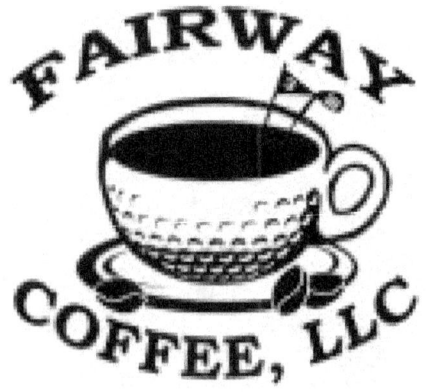

75 cents off purchase of Sunrise Bagel product

75 cents off purchase of Sunrise Bag...

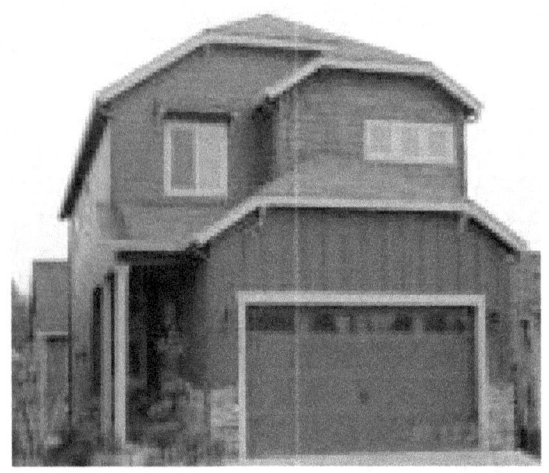

3703 NW 122ND ST Vancouver WA 98685

$296,000 MLS #:14132612 Bedrooms: ...

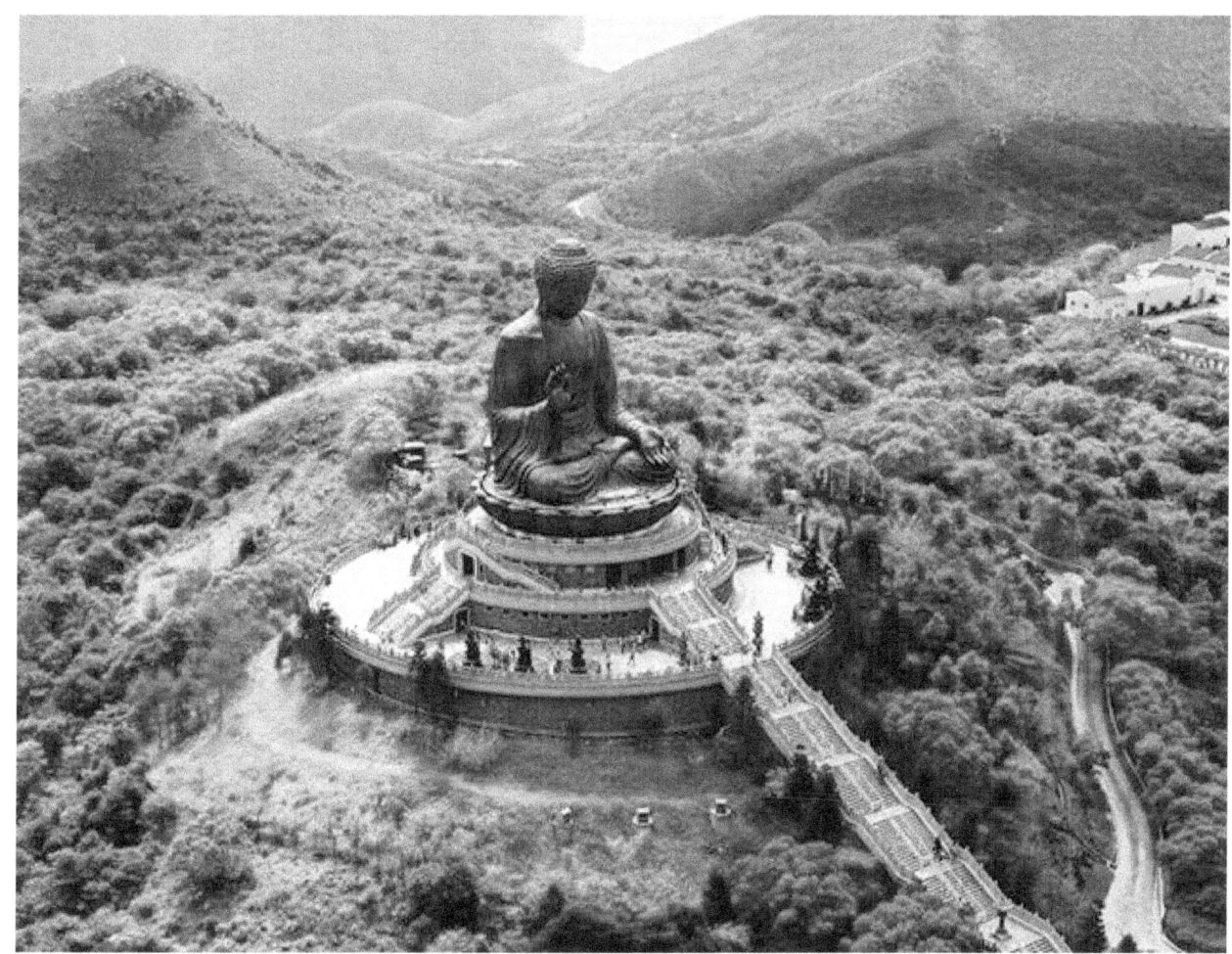

Amazing Place To Visit:

# Lantau Island, Hong Kong: located at the mouth of the <u>Pearl River</u>. Administratively, most of Lantau Island is part of the <u>Islands District</u> of Hong Kong. A small northeastern portion of the island is located in the <u>Tsuen Wan District</u>.

Originally the site of fishing villages, the island has been developed in recent years with the construction of <u>Tung Chung</u> New Town on its north-western coast and the completion of several major infrastructure projects, including<u>Lantau Link</u> (1997), <u>Hong Kong International Airport</u> (1998), <u>Hong Kong Disneyland</u> (2005) and <u>Ngong Ping 360</u> (2006).

# HOW TO USE A SAUNA AND STEAM ROOM PROPERLY

*Using a steam room or a sauna is a beneficial way to relax the muscles, revitalize the skin, improve blood circulation, and ease mental stress. However, due to the extreme heat produced by these facilities, and due to the fact that most spas and saunas are public facilities, all users should take some important safety measures before stepping inside.*

## Step 1

Determine whether the steam room or sauna is co-ed. If it is co-ed, chances are pretty good that the facility will require you to wear a bathing suit. A facility with separate rooms for men and women may establish a bathing suit-optional rule. Either way, it is a good idea to bring a towel and wear sandals into the steam room or sauna in order to shield any bare skin from the hot seating area and also protect it from the sweat produced by other users. Read all signs posted outside the facility before you robe or disrobe.

## Step 2

The heat in steam rooms and saunas causes the body to perspire, often in great amounts. <u>Drink plenty of water before entering in order to combat dehydration</u>. Also shower to remove any lotions or cleansers that are apt to melt or drip off into the facility. Also check your body for any metal (jewelry and zippers, for example) in order to prevent it from burning your body when it quickly heats up in the facility.

## Step 3

Don't remain in the sauna or steam room beyond your own capacity to tolerate the heat. If you begin to feel faint, nauseated, or your heart rate begins to speed, you should exit the sauna or steam room immediately. Generally, to begin with, 8 to 10 minutes in the facility should be enough to cause your body temperature to rise and produce sweat without causing negative physical effects such as dizziness. Take a break and cool off for a little while, and if you feel comfortable returning to the facility, spend another 5 to 10 minutes in there. While in the sauna or steam room, <u>don't mess with any of the controls by pouring water on steamers or adjusting the temperature dials</u>. Speak to an employee if the temperature in the facility doesn't seem warm enough.

## Step 4

Avoid jumping into a cool pool or shower right away. Spend 10 to 15 minutes letting your body adjust to cooler air temperatures in order avoid putting your body through shock when you enter the pool or shower. Drink plenty of water throughout the day to hydrate your body.

## Step 5

Know when not to use facilities. If you are pregnant or think you may be pregnant, abstain from using a steam room or sauna. Raising your body's temperature to that extreme can harm the fetus. Additionally, stay out of the facilities if you have been drinking alcohol or taking illicit drugs. You should also avoid using a sauna or steam room if you are under age 18, if you suffer from circulatory problems, heart disease, high or low blood pressure, diabetes, epilepsy, or any other condition that may affect your body's reaction to high temperatures. Consult a doctor if you believe you may have one of these conditions.

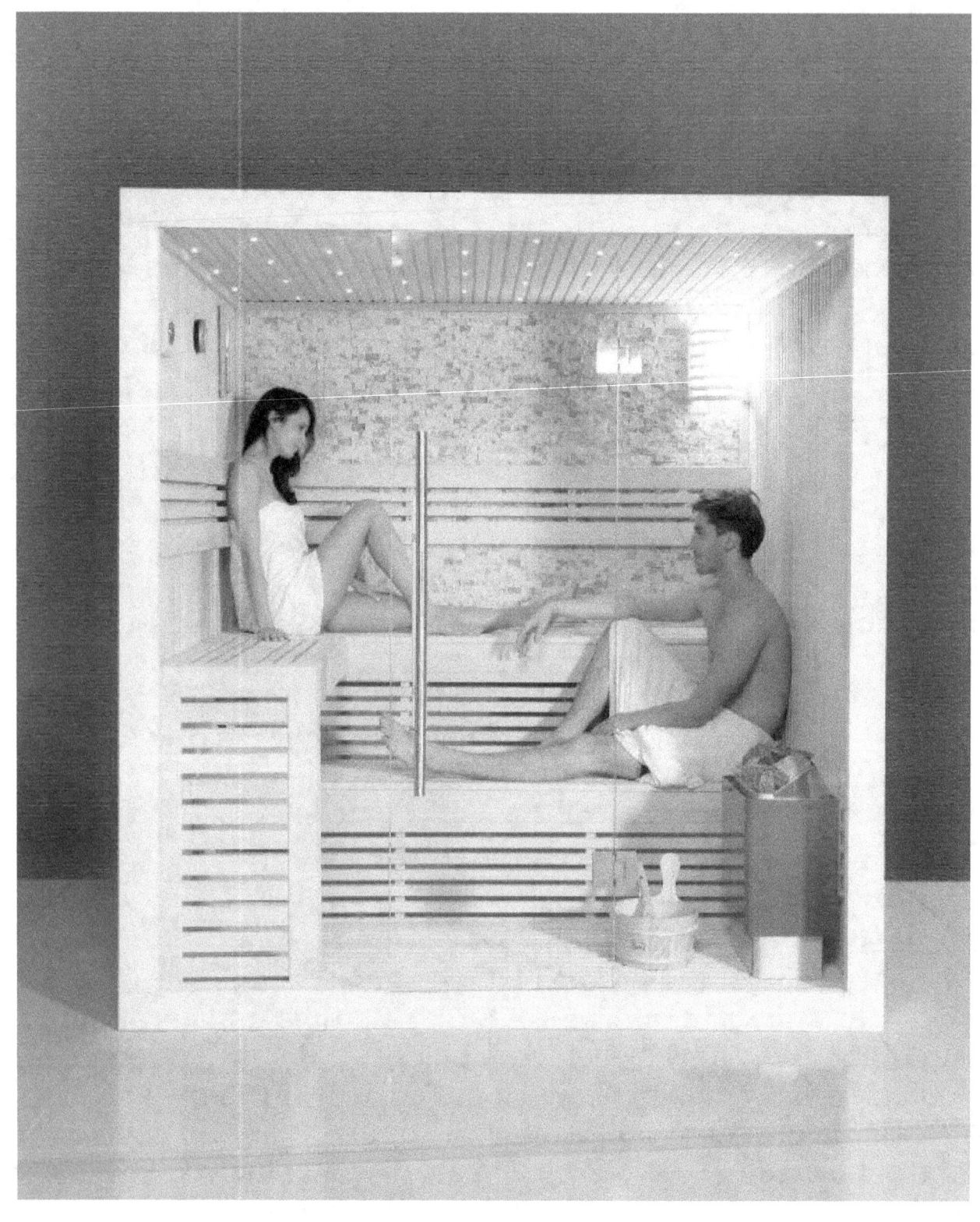

Editing by (Eddie Adel) weconnect2@live.com

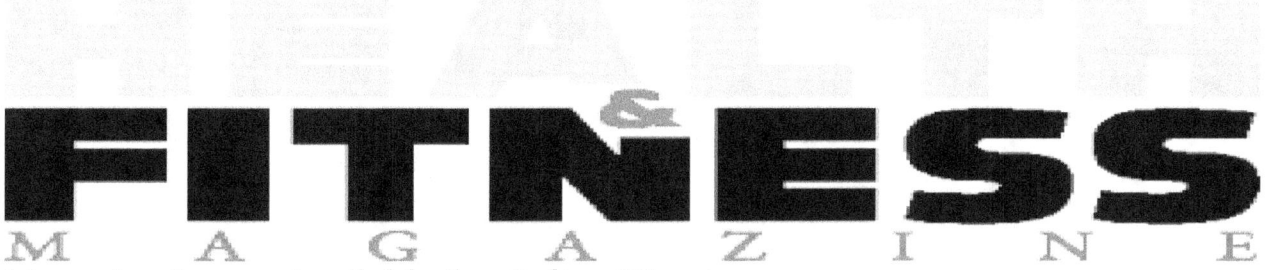

Magazine Issues Available for Online Viewing...Unable to catch our Magazine as it hits the stands? READ the last four issues of our Magazine in all its' glory, in *Adobe Acrobat PDF\** file format. To REA

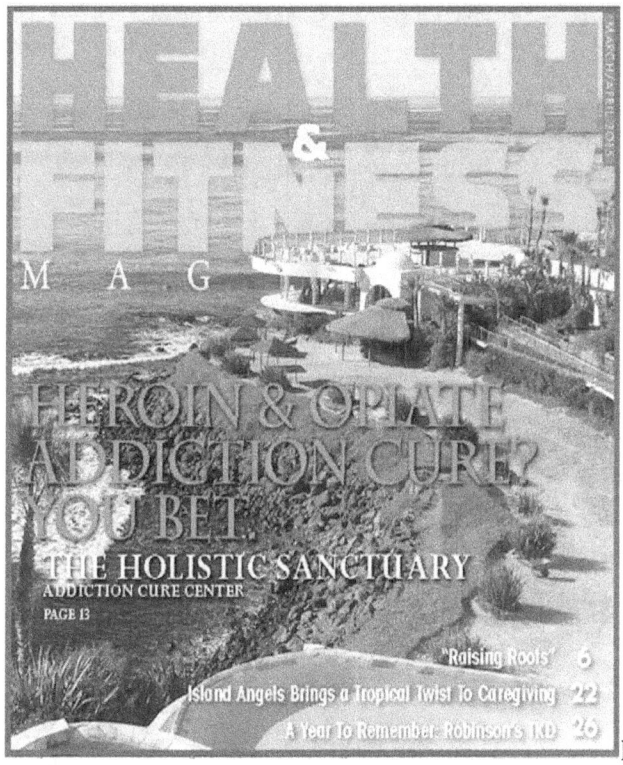

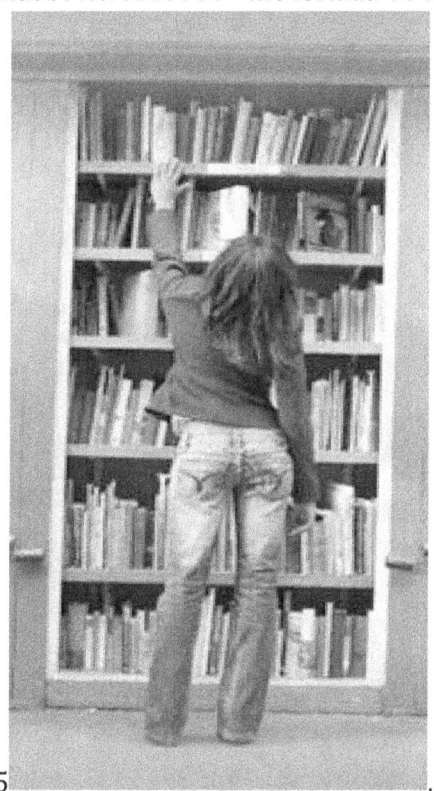

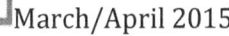

March/April 2015

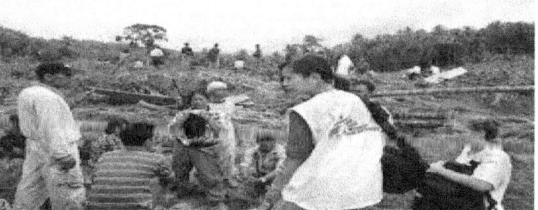

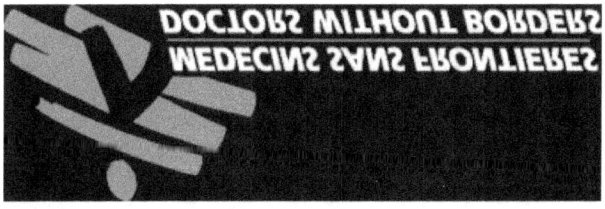

Visit Doctors Without Borders on the web at: http://www.doctorswithoutborders.org/Donate to Doctors Without Borders: https://donate.doctorswithoutborders.org/monthly.cfm